Nair Caetano Domingos
Branca M.O. Santos
Everton Edjar A. Silva

Systemic arterial hypertension from a health promotion perspective

**Nair Caetano Domingos
Branca M.O. Santos
Everton Edjar A. Silva**

Systemic arterial hypertension from a health promotion perspective

Systemic arterial hypertension

ScienciaScripts

Imprint

Any brand names and product names mentioned in this book are subject to trademark, brand or patent protection and are trademarks or registered trademarks of their respective holders. The use of brand names, product names, common names, trade names, product descriptions etc. even without a particular marking in this work is in no way to be construed to mean that such names may be regarded as unrestricted in respect of trademark and brand protection legislation and could thus be used by anyone.

Cover image: www.ingimage.com

This book is a translation from the original published under ISBN 978-613-9-64619-7.

Publisher:
Sciencia Scripts
is a trademark of
Dodo Books Indian Ocean Ltd. and OmniScriptum S.R.L publishing group

120 High Road, East Finchley, London, N2 9ED, United Kingdom
Str. Armeneasca 28/1, office 1, Chisinau MD-2012, Republic of Moldova, Europe
Printed at: see last page
ISBN: 978-620-7-76920-9

I DEDICATE and thank God and Spirituality, who granted me this mission and opportunity, supporting me at all times to fulfil it.

ACKNOWLEDGEMENTS

To my supervisor, Dr Branca Maria de Oliveira Santos, for her trust, collaboration, patience, encouragement and support at various crucial moments, both professional and personal. I would like to thank her for the knowledge she passed on throughout the project, as well as her care and attention. I would like to thank her family, who welcomed me into their home with great joy and affection.

To the participants in this research for the trust they placed in me by opening the doors of their homes and sharing the richness of their experiences with me.

To my niece Clarice Cipriano Domingos, thank you for your example of strength, overcoming, joy, will to live and win. You encouraged me to fight against my fears and difficulties in the search for the truth. I love you!

To my parents João Domingos da Silva and Maria Helena Caetano Domingos, who always encourage the continuous search for knowledge. Thank you for your love, encouragement, support, prayers and trust at all times.

I would like to thank my sister Juçara and my brothers, Vitorino, Marquinho, Renato and Eduardo, my sisters-in-law, brother-in-law and nephews for their encouragement, support and understanding of my absence during the good times and especially the difficult ones. To my niece Bruna, for her care and companionship in the most difficult moments of this journey.

To Ana Terra, Helena, João and Arthur, Auntie's little ones, for their love and joy, making this journey lighter.

To my friend Natália, for her companionship and complicity at all times, in the classroom, at work, for her pleasant company during the long, tiring and risky journeys to Franca. In short, for sharing this whole journey with so much joy. I would like to thank Joelber for solving all the problems I had with my laptops and for his words of encouragement.

Thank you to Amanda, my childhood friend, who welcomed me into her home. Thank you for everything!

To Rosângela, Rodrigo, Keila and Regiene, who are also my family, I thank you for the affection with which you have supported me on this long journey.

I would like to thank the neonatal ICU team for their patience and the physiotherapy team, especially Marco Aurélio, Fernanda, Juliana and Patrícia for their support, guidance and the many changes of duty.

I would like to thank Reinaldinho, who helped me with my English.

I would like to thank the Municipal Health Department of Patos de Minas for allowing this research to take place. The nurses at the health units and all the community health agents, for their guidance on the routine of the service and for their collaboration in the active search for participants, making their time and data available.

To Everton for his availability and help during data collection.

To Prof Dr José Eduardo Zaia, for his suggestions in the dissertation seminar and many other times when I needed them, always so kind and attentive.

To the members of the qualification committee, Dr Wilza Vieira Villela and Dr Paulo Roberto Veiga Quemelo, for their comments and valuable suggestions aimed at enhancing the work.

I would like to thank Jean Ezequiel Limongi for his guidance, affection, education, suggestions and strength to keep going.

To all the colleagues, staff and professors of the Unifran Postgraduate Programme in Health Promotion, who were able to share their teachings with us with competence and dedication.

I would like to thank everyone who contributed directly or indirectly to the completion of this study, and I hope that one day I will be able to repay them.

SUMMARY

DOMINGOS, Nair Caetano. **Systemic arterial hypertension from a health promotion perspective.** 2013. 92 f. Dissertation (Master's in Health Promotion) - University of Franca, Franca.

The aim of this study was to describe the living and health conditions of individuals diagnosed with Systemic Arterial Hypertension (SAH), registered and monitored by the Community Health Agents Programme (PACS) in a municipality in the state of Minas Gerais. The approach chosen was descriptive, cross-sectional research. Data was collected using an interview form. Forty hypertensive patients took part in the study. Of all those interviewed, 57.5% were female, 55.0% were aged between 51 and 60 and 65.0% were married. Of the participants, 55.0% reported blood pressure (BP) levels lower than 140/90 mmHg, 52.5% reported being overweight/obese and 42.5% mentioned being sedentary. Drug treatment was reported by 95.0% of the participants and 57.5% were treated with a combination of two, three or four drugs. Of the total, 50.0% reported a family income of two to three minimum wages and 57.5% were working. There was the same proportion of individuals with complete and incomplete first and second degrees, with 45.0%, respectively. With regard to lifestyle habits, 82.5% reported eating a low-sodium diet and 60.0% reported not drinking alcohol. Most of the interviewees, 62.5%, reported changes in their habits and lifestyle to control their BP. The majority (85.0%) said they had used the public health service for diagnosis and 92.5% were monitoring and treating the disease. Medical appointments were attended every six months by 50.0% of the participants and the initial medical treatment after the diagnosis of hypertension was medication, as reported by 67.5% of the interviewees. Around 55.0% said there were meetings and discussion groups on SAH, although the majority said they didn't take part; 52.5% said they had been monitored by the same health team in 2011, 87.5% said they found no difficulties in monitoring and treating SAH and 50.0% said the care and monitoring provided by the health professionals at their health centre was good. In view of the implications that hypertension has for individuals, knowing the profile of hypertensive patients and the health service provided to them may help to inform discussion and the development of individual and collective actions and decisions within the health system to favour the health and well-being of these individuals, enabling a better prospect of controlling the disease.

Key words: Hypertension; Health Promotion; Primary Health Care, Community Health Agents.

SUMMARY

PRESENTATION

Considering my background in physiotherapy, I have always worked in the care of patients with cardiovascular events, mainly related to systemic arterial hypertension (SAH), both in the acute and chronic phases, in hospitals and emergency care units (UPA), in clinics and at home.

In these professional experiences, I was faced with the presence of varying degrees of sequelae and/or disabilities, some of them permanent, which brought difficulties, suffering and expenses never expected by the family and the patient themselves, culminating in manifestations of stress in the face of possible risks to life and quality of life.

These experiences sparked my interest in researching SAH at home, looking for an approach that not only considered the clinical aspects, based on the biomedical model, with a focus on the disease and drug treatment, but that valued other aspects that make up the determinants of the health-disease process, with a view to clarifying, guiding and showing people that even if you have a chronic disease it is possible to have quality of life.

When I joined the Master's programme in Health Promotion, my concept of health and its determinants was broadened, increasing my understanding that biological, social, economic and/or cultural conditions have a direct influence on the health and quality of life of individuals.

In order to get to know hypertensive individuals, listen to them, find out what their living and health conditions are like, their habits, their desires, needs, difficulties and doubts, and how they are assisted by the health services, I tried to direct the collection instrument following the "Health Field" model, presented by Lalonde in 1974[1], which emphasises the role of four components: human biology, the environment, lifestyle and the organisation of health services, which need to be in balance for the condition of health to be established, allowing for an understanding of the totality of the determining factors of health, in a unifying vision of the health-disease process, highlighting the basic causes, the ways or conditions of life, work and man's relationship with himself, his fellow human beings and the environment.

In view of the implications that hypertension has for individuals, knowing the profile of hypertensive patients in a municipality in the state of Minas Gerais, based on the data related to the four components of this model, will help me to discuss and draw up individual and collective actions and decisions that can favour the health and well-being of these individuals, enabling better control of the disease.

In the course of this study, I present a literature review covering the clinical, epidemiological and social aspects of SAH and the relationship between the disease and Health Promotion. This is followed by the proposed objectives and a description of the theoretical and methodological framework adopted for its development, which will provide orderly and detailed information for its reproducibility. The data obtained will be presented in order to characterise the study population in terms of the four components of the proposed model and compared in the light of the results of other authors concerned with the subject. Finally, conclusions and considerations will be drawn.

CHAPTER 1

INTRODUCTION

1.1   Systemic arterial hypertension: a public health problem.

Systemic arterial hypertension (SAH) or simply arterial hypertension (AH), defined as a multifactorial clinical condition, with high and sustained levels of blood pressure (BP)[2] , is one of the main chronic non-communicable diseases (NCDs) and one of the biggest public health problems in Brazil and worldwide, given the high morbidity and mortality rates related to it and the high cost of its control and treatment[3] . Considered one of the main modifiable risk factors for the development of cardiovascular diseases (CVD), it has a high prevalence and low control rates[4, 5] .

In the last four decades of the last century, Brazil, following the global trend, underwent processes of demographic, epidemiological and nutritional transition that produced an age pyramid with greater relative weight for adults and the elderly, leading to a significant increase in the prevalence of NCDs, with rising estimates of SAH, whose impact on populations will be even more damaging in the coming years[6, 7] .

Although the proportion of the world's population with high BP levels or uncontrolled hypertension decreased modestly between 1980 and 2008, due to population growth and ageing, the number of people with AH increased from 600 million in 1980 to 1.2 billion in 2008[8] .

The global prevalence of AH in 2008 in individuals over 25 years of age was 40 per cent. Grouping countries according to their level of development, it was higher in low and medium development countries, with rates of around 40 per cent for both sexes. In regions of Africa, these figures were close to 46 per cent. In developed countries, the prevalence was 35 per cent for both sexes. Worldwide mortality attributed to AH in 2009 was 7.6 million deaths, around 12.8 per cent of all deaths[2, 8-10] . Globally, SAH is responsible for 62% of strokes and 49% of acute myocardial infarctions (AMI) .[11]

In Brazil, the prevalence of AH varies from 24.8% to 44.4%, due to the different classification criteria and age limits adopted in the surveys. Between the sexes, it is found in 35.8 per cent of men and 30 per cent of women. It affects around 17 million Brazilians and, in the over-60 age group, its prevalence is over 60 per cent. Around 30 per cent of hypertensive patients are unaware of their condition[2, 4, 9] . The financial costs spent on hospitalisations and hospital costs by the Unified Health System (SUS), related to AH and hypertensive diseases, can demand 17.6% of hospitalisations, which corresponds to 5.9% of the resources paid by the SUS[10] .

In 2002-2003, the Ministry of Health (MS) carried out a household survey on risk behaviours and self-reported morbidity of non-communicable diseases and conditions to determine the prevalence of self-reported AH in a population aged over 25 in 15 Brazilian state capitals and the Federal District. The prevalence ranged from 7.4% to 15.7% in people aged between 25 and 39, from 26% to 36.4% in those aged between 40 and 59 and from 39 to 59% in those aged 60 or over[12, 13].

In the state of Minas Gerais, data from a survey carried out by the Ministry of Health in Brazilian state capitals, using the telephone survey for the Surveillance of Risk and Protective Factors for Chronic Diseases (VIGITEL), revealed that the prevalence of AH in the state capital was 22.4 per cent, based on previous medical diagnosis of AH and the amount reported by individuals. In males it was 19.1% and in females 25.3%[14].

The Household Sample Survey Bulletin (PAD-MG), a study that investigated the prevalence of chronic diseases in the state, including AH, through a previous diagnosis of AH given by a doctor or other health professional and reported by individuals in their households, highlighted AH as the most prevalent pathology in the state. When all ages are taken into account, it accounted for 15.7 per cent. In the population aged over 14, the percentage was close to 19.7% and in the elderly population (60 years and over) the figure was approximately 58.3%[15].

Studies on the prevalence and risk factors associated with SAH in Brazil have been carried out more frequently in certain regions, such as the states of São Paulo and Rio Grande do Sul, with high prevalence results. Few studies have been carried out in the state of Minas Gerais and its inland municipalities, which makes it difficult to know the local epidemiological profile. In a study carried out in 2004 in the municipality of Formiga, the prevalence of AH was 32.7%, with 31.7% for males and 33.6% for females. This figure is higher than the values found in a study carried out in the municipality of Bambuí, also in the state, in 1997, with a total prevalence of 24.8%, 26.9% in females and 22.0% in males[16-18].

SAH or AH is often related to functional and/or structural changes in target organs (heart, brain, kidneys and blood vessels) and metabolic changes, with a consequent increase in the risk of fatal and non-fatal cardiovascular events[2, 5]. The asymptomatic nature of SAH prevents its early detection. Known as a silent disease, it progressively damages target organs and must be monitored regularly in order to be detected and treated early.[19]

Hypertension is classified into two main groups. The first, called Primary Hypertension (PH), essential or idiopathic, accounts for 90 to 95 per cent of cases and no specific cause can be identified[19, 20]. In general, individuals with this type of hypertension have easily identifiable behaviours: excessive consumption of calories, salt or alcohol, which can be associated with smoking, risk factors that contribute to an increase in BP.[19]

In the second group, called Secondary Systemic Arterial Hypertension (SAH), the prevalence is between 5 and 10 per cent. This arises from a known pathology and is therefore secondary to it[20, 21]. The causes can be renal, vascular, endocrine or neurogenic. Regardless of the origin of hypertension, the final common denominator is a sustained increase in peripheral vascular resistance.[19, 21]

AH is diagnosed by detecting high and sustained levels of BP measured by doctors of any speciality and other health professionals. This diagnosis is validated by repeated measurements in the doctor's office, under ideal conditions, on at least three occasions. Measurements should be taken from both upper limbs, positioned at heart level, preferably in a sitting position and, in the event of a difference in the values found, the result with the highest value is used as the reference[2, 22] .

The classification of BP into normal and high values is always a moving target[19] . For the Brazilian Society of Cardiology, ideal or optimal values for individuals over the age of 18 are arterial pressures lower than 120-129 mmHg for systolic blood pressure (SBP) and 80-84 mmHg for diastolic blood pressure (DBP), so that the individual presents the lowest cardiovascular risk[2] .

Pre-hypertension is defined as slightly increased blood pressure, considering SBP values between 130-139 mmHg and DBP values between 85-89 mmHg. AH is classified into stages 1, 2, 3 and isolated systolic hypertension. Between 140-159 mmHg for SBP and 90-99 mmHg for DBP is considered stage 1; between 160-179 mmHg (SBP) and 100-109 mmHg (DBP), stage 2; in stage 3 SBP is greater than or equal to ($\geq$) 180 mmHg *and* DBP $\geq$ 110 mmHg. Isolated systolic hypertension is defined as SBP > 140 mmHg and DBP less than 90 mmHg[2] .

The dividing line that defines hypertension is SBP $\geq$ 140 mmHg and/or DBP $\geq$ 90 mmHg. Clinical studies show that mortality from CVD increases progressively as BP rises from 115/75 mmHg in a linear, continuous and independent manner[2, 23, 24] .

The main risk factors that favour the development of AH are classified as non-modifiable: heredity, gender, age, race and modifiable: sedentary lifestyle, stress, smoking, high sodium and fat diet, obesity and alcohol consumption[24, 25] . Thus, due to its close correlation with lifestyle, AH can be prevented, minimised or treated by adopting healthy lifestyle habits[26] .

The overall prevalence of SAH between the sexes is similar, although it is higher in men up to the age of 50 and in women after that age. With regard to race, it is twice as prevalent in non-white individuals. Brazilian studies with a simultaneous approach to gender and colour have shown a predominance of non-white women with AH of up to 130% compared to white women. The exact impact of miscegenation on hypertension in Brazil is unknown[2] .

Age has a direct and linear relationship with hypertension. It is an important risk factor for its development due to the transformations typical of ageing, with changes in the smooth muscle and connective tissue of the vessels[2, 5, 9] .

The development of hypertension is facilitated by an unhealthy lifestyle, which includes high sodium and low potassium intake, excessive alcohol consumption, high calorific intake and physical inactivity. The last two risk factors are the ones that most contribute to the development of excess weight and obesity, which are directly related to the rise in BP[27] .

Generally, hypertension does not occur in isolation. It is not uncommon for hypertensive individuals to have associated metabolic abnormalities, such as obesity, insulin resistance and dyslipidaemia, which is referred to as Cardiovascular Metabolic Syndrome. It significantly increases cardiovascular risk and requires aggressive intervention for each specific risk factor[2, 21].

A sedentary lifestyle acts as a predisposing factor for increased BP due to its close relationship with weight gain. Physical activity reduces the incidence of hypertension, even in pre-hypertensive individuals. It contributes significantly to the control and reduction of hypertension, as it results in a decrease of at least 10 to 20 mmHg in resting BP, as a consequence of the reduction in body weight, and is indicated for both the prevention and treatment of hypertension[2, 19].

The daily sodium requirement for humans is that contained in 5 grams (g) of sodium chloride or table salt, i.e. 2 g of sodium. Daily salt intake should be reduced to 5g in controlled hypertension and 2g in severe hypertension. The average Brazilian consumes twice as much as recommended by the World Health Organisation (WHO), which states that the nutritional requirement for sodium in human beings is 500 mg, about 1.2 g of table salt[27- 29]. Normotensive individuals with high sensitivity to sodium intake have a five times higher incidence of raising their BP and developing into hypertension over a 15-year period when compared to individuals with low sensitivity. Despite individual differences in sensitivity, even small reductions in the amount of salt are effective in reducing BP[2].

The daily intake of potassium should be between 2 and 4 g, contained in a diet rich in fresh fruit and vegetables. Increasing potassium intake prevents a rise in BP and preserves cerebral circulation, preventing stroke[28].

Daily consumption of alcohol in high doses raises BP levels and blood pressure variability, increases the prevalence of hypertension and is one of the causes of resistance to antihypertensive therapy. Individuals who have a daily habit of drinking alcoholic beverages should be advised not to exceed 30g of ethanol a day for men and half that amount for women, and preferably to drink it sporadically[2, 30].

Smoking has a cholinergic effect on the central nervous system through its main agent: nicotine. It promotes the release of catecholamines, adrenaline, vasopressin and other hormones that trigger an increase in heart rate and peripheral vascular resistance, resulting in an increase in BP. Smoking contributes to resistance to the effect of antihypertensive drugs and stopping smoking is a priority measure in the primary and secondary prevention of cardiovascular diseases[2, 27, 31].

There is evidence linking psychosocial stress with AH related to "stressful conditions", such as social dissatisfaction, low educational level, unemployment, and especially those professional activities characterised by high psychological demands and poor control of these situations[27].

Investigations of the clinical and laboratory history help with the diagnosis, aetiology and treatment of hypertension. In these interventions, special attention should be paid to relevant data such as risk factors, diabetes mellitus (DM), signs of secondary hypertension and target organ damage. In this assessment it is also important to consider family and socio-economic aspects and the individual's lifestyle characteristics[2, 27, 28].

The basic laboratory assessment includes tests that investigate clinical lesions in target organs and risk factors for developing AH, CVD and comorbidities. This should include urine tests, creatinine and serum potassium, fasting glycaemia, total cholesterol, HDL, triglycerides, uric acid and a resting electrocardiogram[27].

Cardiovascular risk stratification is essential for establishing the treatment of hypertension and its prognosis, as it determines the likelihood of a serious cardiovascular event occurring in the next ten years[2, 25, 28]. Five categories of absolute cardiovascular risk are defined: baseline risk, low additional risk, moderate additional risk, high additional risk and very high additional risk, showing that even patients classified as hypertensive in stages 1, 2 or 3 can belong to categories of greater or lesser risk depending on comorbidities or associated risk factors[2, 28].

The baseline and low additional risk group includes men under 55 years of age and women 65 years of age, with normal, borderline or stage 1 BP, including a maximum of two risk factors. In these individuals, the probability of a serious cardiovascular event in the next 10 years is less than 15%[2, 25].

The moderate additional risk group includes individuals with low BP levels but associated with three or more risk factors, who may have target organ damage, DM and/or metabolic syndrome; while other individuals have high BP levels and no or at most two associated risk factors. The probability of a serious cardiovascular event in this group is between 15 and 20 per cent[2, 25].

In the additional high risk group, the probability of a cardiovascular event is 20 to 30 per cent. This group includes pre-hypertensive individuals, stage 1 and 2 hypertensive individuals with three or more risk factors, who may have target organ damage, DM and/or metabolic syndrome, and some stage 3 hypertensive individuals with no associated risk factors[2, 25].

Finally, the very high additional risk group are normotensive, pre-hypertensive and stage 1, 2 and 3 hypertensive patients, who have more than one risk factor associated with comorbidities such as DM, target organ damage, metabolic syndrome, manifest cardiovascular or kidney disease. The probability of a cardiovascular event in the next ten years is greater than 30 per cent. For this group, immediate and effective drug therapy is indicated[2, 25, 28].

The decision to treat AH is based on the BP levels and cardiovascular risk stratification obtained during the clinical assessment[2, 25, 27]. The choice of treatment must take into account the presence of risk factors and concomitant diseases such as diabetes, obesity, target organ damage (TOD), kidney disease and cardiovascular disease. This includes strategies such as education and guidance on changing lifestyle habits, whether or not associated with drug therapy[2, 28]. Pharmacological treatment aims to reduce BP, but its primary objective is to reduce the cardiovascular morbidity and mortality of hypertensive patients[2, 32].

For hypertensive patients with low cardiovascular risk, the recommended time period for lifestyle changes alone, i.e. non-drug therapy, is a maximum of six months. These changes can delay or prevent the development of hypertension in individuals with borderline blood pressure. This individual should be re-evaluated no later than six months after starting non-drug treatment, to confirm that BP has been controlled. If this benefit is not confirmed, drug treatment in combination with non-drug treatment is indicated[2]. In the presence of heart failure, renal failure or DM, even with low blood pressures, immediate drug treatment should be started[27].

In hypertensive patients with medium, high or very high cardiovascular risk, drug therapy should be instituted promptly in all individuals, regardless of BP. The aim of this early initiation is to reduce the impact of high BP and to protect target organs. The approach should be combined, drug and non-drug therapy, in order to achieve the recommended goal as early as possible[2, 25].

The targets for BP values to be achieved are: for stage 1 and 2 hypertensive patients with low and medium cardiovascular risk, BP < 140/90; for hypertensive and pre-hypertensive patients with high cardiovascular risk, BP < 130/85; and very high cardiovascular risk BP < 130/80 and, finally, nephropathic hypertensive patients with proteinuria > 1.0g/l, BP < 120/75. If the individual tolerates the treatment, it is recommended to achieve lower BP values than those indicated as minimum targets, reaching, if possible, values ≤ 120/80, pressure levels considered optimal[2].

When starting drug treatment, hypertensive patients should be explained the probable adverse effects, the possibility of any changes to the therapy and the time needed for the full effect of the drugs to be achieved. Currently, the groups of antihypertensive drugs commercially available in Brazil are divided into classes: 1 diuretics (Hydrochlorothiazide / Furosemide); direct vasodilators (Minoxidil / Hydralazine); calcium channel antagonists or blockers (Verapamil / Nifedipine); angiotensin-converting enzyme inhibitors (Captopril / Enalapril); angiotensin II AT^1 receptor blockers (Losartan / Valsartan); direct renin inhibitors (Aliskiren); adrenergic inhibitors, which are classified into three groups: centrally acting inhibitors (Alfamethyldopa / Clonidine), beta-blockers (Atenolol / Propanolol) and alpha-blockers (Doxazosin / Prazosin)[2]. Only examples of the most commonly used drugs by class have been cited.

Monotherapy can be used as an initial antihypertensive strategy in patients with stage 1 hypertension and low to moderate cardiovascular risk. However, when BP cannot be controlled with a single drug, it is necessary to use combination therapy, which can be from the same or different groups, especially in individuals with high and very high cardiovascular risk, diabetics and comorbidities[2, 24, 32].

Although pharmacological treatment is the foundation for clinical treatment, individuals should be continually encouraged to adopt healthy lifestyle habits such as losing and maintaining adequate weight, practising regular physical activity, stopping smoking, reducing the consumption of fat, salt and alcoholic drinks. Even if these interventions do not produce a significant reduction in BP to avoid drug therapy in individuals known to be hypertensive, they do reduce the number of drugs or dosages needed for control[20, 24, 28].

Non-drug treatment, which requires lifestyle changes, is indicated for all hypertensive patients, regardless of the stage or severity of the disease, as a form of health promotion[2, 27]. Changes in lifestyle habits can be achieved with constant encouragement during consultations and guidance throughout follow-up by the doctor and his team. For the treatment to be effective, it is of fundamental importance that the patient is well orientated and actively involved[19, 28] . Making changes is slow, painful and involves educational measures that require continuity in their implementation[27] .

Educational activities should include information on the causes and consequences of untreated or poorly controlled AH, reinforcing the importance of continuous use of medication, proper nutrition as an essential part of treatment, dispelling myths, insecurities and anxiety, emphasising the benefits of physical activity and providing guidance on healthy lifestyle habits. Ongoing counselling and education is a fundamental part of the treatment of hypertension and is the right of the individual and the duty of those responsible for health promotion[28] .

1.2 Health promotion as a strategy for the prevention and control of systemic arterial hypertension

SAH or simply arterial hypertension (AH), as a chronic condition, initially asymptomatic, with a high prevalence and high social cost, with a major impact on the morbidity and mortality profile of the Brazilian and world population, has represented a challenge for public health systems, even though it is avoidable and preventable[2, 3] . Some strategies can be used to minimise its onset and the resulting complications, including early detection, encouraging physical activity, reducing smoking and restricting excessive consumption of unhealthy foods. This prevention should be aimed for and carried out at the different levels of health care[33] .

Health Promotion (HP) was referred to when the Natural History of Disease Model was developed in its three levels of prevention: primary, which covers the pre-pathogenesis period and includes health promotion and specific protection; secondary, which covers the beginning of pathogenesis and includes diagnosis, early treatment and limiting disability; and tertiary, which occurs when complications and disability have already set in, through rehabilitation. The concept of PH in primary prevention, as a measure aimed at increasing health and general well-being[34-37] has been changing over the last 25 years, with new currents of promotion emerging, especially in Canada, the USA and Western European countries[37] .

In 1974, the modern health promotion movement began in Canada with the publication of the document "A new perspective on the health of Canadians", better known as the Lalonde Report, the first official document to use the term health promotion. This document was produced out of political, technical and economic motivation, aimed at tackling the high costs in the health sector due to exclusively medical care for chronic diseases, with unsatisfactory results[36] .

Using the "Field of Health" model, which brings together the so-called "determinants of health", the document breaks down this field and groups it into four categories, in perfect balance and importance: human biology, the environment, lifestyle and the organisation of health care[1] . Simultaneously with the emergence of the Lalonde Report on the world stage, underpinning the discussions of the First International Conference on HP, non-communicable diseases also emerged as a Public Health problem in almost all countries, and the actions used by health systems to combat them were almost all geared towards medical care, which did not show good results in terms of cost and effectiveness[38] .

Thus, primary health care, which was born as an idea in the 70s, began to be referenced in official documents and consolidated in the 80s. In this process, the WHO played a leading role, promoting events, issuing publications or encouraging debate on the principles, concepts and strategies of HP around the world, such as the First International Conference on Primary Health Care in Alma-Ata in 1978 and the First International Conference on Health Promotion in 1986 in Ottawa, Canada, which culminated in the drafting of the Ottawa Charter. Today, in fact, there is no way of thinking about HP without referring to the WHO[35, 36, 39] .

According to the Ottawa Charter, HP is the name given to the process of empowering the community to act to improve its quality of life and health, including greater participation in controlling this process. To achieve a state of physical, mental and social well-being, individuals and groups must be able to identify aspirations, satisfy needs and favourably modify the environment. Thus, HP is not the sole responsibility of the health sector, but goes beyond a healthy lifestyle towards global well-being[40] .

The Ottawa Charter still remains the centrepiece of the HP strategy, and its concepts and practices are implemented in health systems and academic spaces around the world[41] . It has guided other conferences, especially when it emphasises the social dimension and the importance of five fundamental strategies for achieving full health: public policy, a healthy environment, strengthening community action, developing personal skills and reorienting the health service .[37, 42]

In Brazil, ideas about HP were introduced in the mid-1980s, fuelled by the debate around Health Reform. The discussion of these ideas was highlighted at the 8th National Health Conference in 1986, where the concepts and objectives of Brazilian society were very similar to those proposed by the 1st International Conference on Health Promotion in Ottawa, Canada, in the same year. It also had an important influence on the First International Conference on Primary Health Care in Alma-Ata (1978), which determined and defended the theme: "Health for all by the year 2000", fomenting the debate around Health Reform.The final reports of these meetings defined health not only as the absence of disease, but conceived of it in broader terms, taking into account other basic needs, including an environment conducive to growth and development and the search for the full realisation of human potential[43, 44] .

The Unified Health System (SUS) was created in Brazil in 1990 in an attempt to organise the health service. It is the greatest achievement of Brazilian society in the field of health and social policies, and a milestone in the country's health history. It is based on three basic principles: universality, equity and comprehensiveness, with a view to guaranteeing every Brazilian citizen the right to health[45] . It was created by the 1988 Federal Constitution and regulated by Laws 8080/90 (Organic Health Law) and 8142/90, with the aim of changing the situation of inequality in health care for the population, making public care compulsory and free for all citizens[46] .

In 1997, when the process of consolidating and decentralising SUS resources began, the Community

Health Agents Programme (PACS), which had been in existence since the early 1990s, was effectively instituted and regulated[41, 47]. PACS institutionalised the experiences of health practices with community agents, which had already been developing in an isolated and focused way in various regions of the country, mainly in the states of Paraná, Mato Grosso do Sul and Ceará, becoming a state policy[48]. Its central aim was to help reduce infant mortality and maternal mortality, with a view to implementing cost-effective basic actions as a way of extending health service coverage to poorer and more disadvantaged areas. Thanks to the recognised success of the programme, the Ministry of Health itself realised that the agents could also be an important part of organising the Basic Health Service in the municipalities[41, 47, 49].

The development of PACS actions is the responsibility of a minimum health team, made up of a doctor, a nurse and six community health agents, who represent a link between the community and the health system, strengthening and creating new links between society and the team[47, 49, 50]. Through visits to families in the community, the agents carry out work aimed at improving the quality of life of the families included in the programme, through the development and implementation of actions aimed at disease prevention and health promotion.[50]

The community health agent (ACS) has the task and routine, among others, of visiting each family in their community or micro-area at least once a month; tracking down information on each member of the family they assist, regarding variables that influence their health and quality of life, registering them on the Household Registration Form - Form A (Annex A) in the Primary Care Information System (SIAB) and referring specific problems to a nurse. The activities carried out by the health agents are monitored and guided by a nurse based at the health unit, who acts as an instructor-supervisor and is also responsible for training the health agents[47].

Later, in a context of restructuring, qualification and expansion of Primary Health Care, the Ministry of Health remodelled and transformed the PACS into the Family Health Programme (PSF), i.e. today it is understood as a transitional strategy for the PSF[41, 47]. The PACS and PSF strategies have significantly expanded access to primary care, the gateway to the health system, with prevention and health promotion as a priority[3].

By prioritising primary care, PACS and PSF represent a strategy to reverse the current way of providing health care, which has always favoured hospital treatment, with a proposal to reorganise primary care and reorient the care model. They are characterised by their alignment with the principles of universality, decentralisation, equity of care, comprehensive actions and community participation, which must be followed so that health actions take place despite the difficulties of the local reality[51, 52].

Implementing these principles of intervention in the prevention of AH represents a major challenge for health managers and professionals. In Brazil, around 75 per cent of the population's healthcare is provided through the public health system (SUS). Primary prevention and early diagnosis of AH, together with effective care, adequate monitoring and establishing links with basic health units, are essential elements for the successful control of this condition and should be the priority goals of health professionals, preventing complications, reducing the number of hospital admissions and mortality, thus promoting health[33, 53] .

In an evolutionary process, in 2001 - 2003, with the aim of reducing cases of morbidity and mortality due to hypertension and diabetes mellitus, the Ministry of Health implemented the Plan to Reorganise Primary Care for Hypertension and Diabetes Mellitus throughout Brazil[12, 33, 54] . A number of actions were implemented in the states and municipalities, including training multipliers to update professionals working in primary care; screening and registration campaigns for hypertensive and diabetic patients and the promotion of healthy lifestyle habits; the promotion of efficient conditions for the diagnosis of AH and DM, and the initiation of therapy; agreeing standards and targets between the three spheres of health management, the inclusion of the National Pharmaceutical Assistance Programme for AH and DM concomitant with the implementation of "Hiperdia", a national computerised system for registering and monitoring hypertensive and diabetic patients in basic health units, and evaluating the impact of the Plan for Reorganising Basic Care for Arterial Hypertension and Diabetes Mellitus[7, 33, 53] .

According to the Ministry of Health, primary care prioritises the prevention and control of hypertension and DM, with educational actions to control risk factors such as obesity, sedentary lifestyles, smoking and the prevention of possible sequelae. Actions such as actively seeking out cases of hypertension, early diagnosis, registration and appropriate treatment are priorities for primary care in the SUS[3] .

It is also worth considering the publication in 2006 of the National Health Promotion Policy (PNPS) and the Strengthening of Primary Care as a priority for the Family Health Strategy, in the qualification of primary care professionals through continuing education, in guaranteeing the infrastructure of Basic Health Units and their financing by the three management spheres of SUS (55)..

CHAPTER 2

1.1   General objective

To describe the living and health conditions of individuals with a medical diagnosis of SAH, registered and monitored by the Community Health Agents Programme (PACS) in a municipality in the state of Minas Gerais.

1.2   Specific objectives

- Describe human biology data related to health, risk factors and complications resulting from SAH;
- Describe the environmental data related to the socioeconomic conditions of individuals with SAH;
- To identify the lifestyle and how individuals with SAH take care of their health;
- Learn about the difficulties, problems and expectations regarding treatment and monitoring of the disease by the health service.

CHAPTER 3

METHOD

3.1 Nature of the study

This is a descriptive, cross-sectional study on the living and health conditions, risk factors, difficulties, complications and expectations faced by individuals with SAH registered and monitored by the PACS in a municipality in Minas Gerais.

The main objective of descriptive research is to describe the characteristics of a particular population or phenomenon. One of its most important characteristics is the use of specific instruments for data collection (questionnaire, interview or form) and, in general, it is the type of research usually carried out by researchers concerned with practical action[56] .

3.2 Study site

The municipality of the study is located in the centre-west region of the state, called Alto Paranaíba, 400 km from the capital (**Figure 1**), with a territorial area of 3,189.771 km² and approximately 139,849 thousand inhabitants, with a Municipal Human Development Index (HDI 2010) of 0.765[57, 58] .

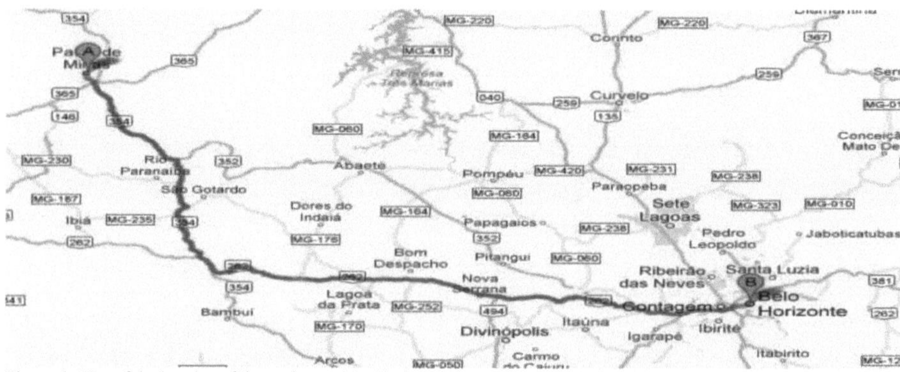

Figure 1: Map of the location of the study municipality in relation to the capital Belo Horizonte.
Source:http://maps. google.com.br

Its main economic activities come from agribusiness and agroindustry. Agriculture is highly diversified, with grain and fruit and vegetable production. Cattle farming is of significant economic and social importance to the municipality. With 442 industries and 2,108

commercial establishments, the municipality accounts for 0.38% of the state's collection of the Tax on the Circulation of Goods and Services (ICMS). Added to other revenues, it ranks 19th in the overall collection of

18

the state of Minas Gerais[59] .

The municipality has five hospitals: one public, i.e. with exclusive Unified Health System (SUS) services, and four private, two of which also have SUS services. These hospitals offer medium and high complexity services, such as haemodialysis, abdominal, thoracic, cardiac, neurological and orthopaedic surgeries, and oncology services. The municipality also has an Emergency Care Unit (UPA), a Psychosocial Care Centre (CAPS), a Viva Vida Centre, a Hiperdia Centre, a Mobile Emergency Care Service (SAMU), two Exceptional Medication Pharmacies and the Popular Pharmacy Programme, a Communicable Disease Care Centre, a Dental Specialities Centre, an Association of Parents and Friends of the Exceptional (APAE) and a Fire Brigade[60, 61] .

In 2000, the municipality set up the Community Health Agents Programme (PACS) and the Family Health Programme (PSF). Currently, the municipality has four PACS and 30 PSFs in 30 Primary Health Care Units (UAPS), with four units running both programmes concurrently (PACS and PSF). The PACS health units are distributed in the Sebastião Amorim I, Guanabara, Jardim Paraíso and Ipanema neighbourhoods[62] , as shown in Figure 2.

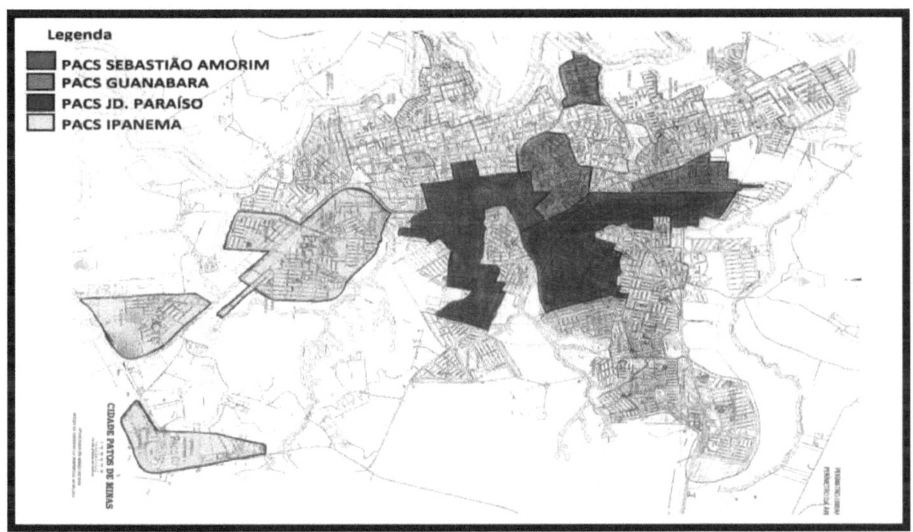

Figure 2: Map of the distribution of PACS in the study municipality
Source: Patos de Minas Municipal Health Department, 2013.
3.2. 1Delimitation of the data collection field

According to 2011 data from the Municipal Health Department[62] , since PACS was set up in the municipality in 2000, 4,369 hypertensive patients have been registered in the four units.

The Sebastião Amorim I neighbourhood health unit is a reference point for approximately 6,713 inhabitants, 720 of whom have been registered with SAH. It covers 12 micro-areas in the Boa Vista, Eldorado, part of Centro and part of Cônego Getúlio neighbourhoods.

19

The Guanabara neighbourhood unit is a reference point for approximately 11,006 inhabitants and has 1,239 registered SAH patients. It covers 14 micro-areas in the Copacabana, Guanabara, part of Centro and Sobradinho neighbourhoods.

The Jardim Paraíso neighbourhood unit is a reference point for approximately 12,105 inhabitants, of whom 1,393 have been registered with SAH. It covers 16 micro-areas in the neighbourhoods of Alto Caiçaras, Caiçaras, Aurélio Caixeta, São Francisco, Vila Garcia, Jardim Floresta, Jardim Centro, Jardim Califórnia and Val Paraíso.

Finally, the Ipanema neighbourhood unit is a reference point for approximately 10,750 inhabitants, has 1,017 registered SAH patients and covers 18 micro areas in the Ipanema, Planalto, Jardim Céu Azul, Gramado, Jardim Peluzzo, Jardim do Andrades, Distrito Industrial I and II neighbourhoods.

All these health units provide care from Monday to Friday, from 7am to 6pm, in three medical specialities (general practice, paediatrics and gynaecology), with a doctor for each speciality and a nurse responsible for each unit. In addition to this team, there are 60 community health agents (ACS), who are responsible for the 60 micro-areas. These agents make monthly home visits, carrying out the activities laid down by the MoH[47] . When necessary, they are accompanied by a doctor and/or nurse from the unit responsible for the micro-areas.

Hypertensive patients are monitored every six months by the nurse, who assesses data relating to BP, heart rate, lower limb oedema and possible complaints related to the disease (headache, chest pain, dizziness). The result of this assessment determines whether or not a referral for medical assessment is necessary. At the end of the service, the patient receives a new prescription for the medication, which is valid for six months.

With the exception of the PACS in the Ipanema neighbourhood, the other health units don't offer any continuing education activities (meetings, groups, lectures) for hypertensive patients. Only the Ipanema neighbourhood unit offers an annual Health Day by the PACS team, with the participation of guest speakers from other areas, such as physiotherapists, physical educators and nutritionists, with a view to continuing health education on the importance of hypertension.
and lifestyle changes. On this day, hypertensive patients are re-evaluated by the nurses and doctors, who request tests for control. The unit also has a Nutritionist Group, which meets with hypertensive patients once a month to advise on diet and monitor data such as weight and waist circumference.

Medicines for registered hypertensive patients are dispensed by the Municipal Pharmacy, where anyone can pick them up as long as they present their prescription, which is valid for six months. The medicines are distributed every two months.

Follow-up of people with hypertension in health units follows a programme run by the Minas Gerais State Health Department - Guidelines for Adult Health Care: Hypertension and Diabetes[25] , defined according to cardiovascular risk stratification. Thus, low-risk hypertensive patients are offered one medical consultation/year, one nursing consultation/year and, depending on the coverage of the area covered by the health agent, one visit/month. An electrocardiogram (ECG) is offered every three years.

For those at medium, high and very high risk, what varies is the number of nursing appointments (three appointments/year for those at medium risk and one appointment/year for those at high and very high risk).

For medium-risk hypertensive patients, an ECG can be requested once a year, and for high- and very high-risk patients, twice every three years. Specialised consultations with cardiologists and/or nephrologists are determined and referred at the doctor's discretion.

Laboratory tests are carried out according to the risk stratification of individuals with SAH. Assessments of serum glucose, creatinine, potassium, cholesterol, triglycerides and urine routine are requested for low-risk individuals, one test every two years, and for medium, high and very high risk individuals, one test per year.

1.3 Research subjects

Although the Primary Care Information System (SIAB) reported 1,197 hypertensive patients registered with the four PACS in 2011[62] , the data proved to be out of date and inconsistent with reality, since when trying to delimit the stratified sample of participants by PACS, one unit was found to have no records of registrations in that year.

In view of this situation, an active search was carried out for hypertensive patients registered with the four PACS, through a search of the household registration forms **(Appendix A)**, which yielded a total number of hypertensive patients.

of 243 hypertensive patients registered in 2011. Of these, 86 were registered with PACS Guanabara, 63 with PACS Sebastião Amorim I, 59 with PACS Jardim Paraíso and 35 with PACS Ipanema.

From this total, a sample was established based on the following inclusion criteria:
- were registered and monitored by PACS as hypertensive in 2011;
- of both sexes (women could not be pregnant);
- aged between 18 and 60;
- be an urban resident;
- agreed to take part in the study by signing the Free and Informed Consent Form **(Appendix A).**

Thus, of the 243 hypertensive patients registered with the PACS in 2011, 120 were excluded because they were under 18 and over 60, leaving 123 individuals. Of these, a further 38 hypertensive patients who were registered but not followed up by the PACS (because they had private health insurance) were excluded, leaving 85 hypertensive patients who made up the study sample, represented by 26 from the Sebastião Amorim I PACS, 24 from the Guanabara PACS, 18 from the Jardim Paraíso PACS and 17 from the Ipanema PACS.

It is worth noting, however, that of the 85 hypertensive patients who met the inclusion criteria for the study, 45 were excluded: 18 (40.0%) because it was impossible to contact them at home after three unsuccessful attempts at different times and on different dates, 18 (40.0%) because they could not be found at the address given on the registration forms and 9 (20.0%) because they refused the invitation to take part in the study.

The sample thus consisted of 40 hypertensive patients, considering that more than one individual per household could take part in the study.

The age group selected between 18 and 60 was chosen in accordance with Law no. 8.069, of 13 July 1990, which provides for the Statute of the Child and Adolescent, where in Art. 2, adolescence is considered to be up to eighteen years of age and in the Statute of the Elderly, Law no.° 10.741, of 1 October 2003, in Art. 1, people aged sixty or over are considered elderly[63, 64].

1.4   Data collection procedure

1.4.1   Preliminary activities

In order to carry out the study, prior contact was made with the municipality's Municipal Health Department, with a view to obtaining consent to carry out the study (**Annex B**).

After approval, an average of six meetings were held with the nurses and CHWs of the respective PACS, when information about the objectives of the study was provided, obtaining their cooperation in providing the identification data of hypertensive individuals (name, age, address and/or telephone number) contained in the household registration forms (**Annex A**) standardised by the Ministry of Health[65].

1.4.2   Data collection instrument

In order to achieve the proposed objectives, an Interview Form (**Appendix B**) was drawn up for data collection, with closed and open questions, adapted for individuals with SAH, structured into five parts, namely: identification data and data related to the four components of the Health Field model[1]: data on human biology, the environment, lifestyle and the organisation of health services. This instrument was developed based on other instruments developed by authors who have used the framework for their research[66-68] and based on the literature related to SAH.

1.4.3   Instrument evaluation

With the aim of evaluating the data collection instrument in order to meet the proposed objectives, it was previously analysed by three judges with recognised expertise in the field of SAH and primary health care (two doctors and a nurse) for its comprehensiveness, content, clarity, objectivity, relevance, accuracy of information and adequacy and reduction of possible doubts that could compromise the collection. The result of this evaluation culminated in the reformulation and removal of questions in order to make the form more objective and less extensive (without jeopardising the achievement of the objectives).

The instrument was then pre-tested by the researcher during a home visit to 12 hypertensive individuals being monitored at the four health centres (three individuals/unit), chosen from the list of the study sample, starting with the first on the list, every three years. If the selected individual refused to take part, they were replaced by the one immediately below them on the list.

The pre-test was carried out in order to assess the operability of the instrument and to detect possible changes and additions. It took an average of 30 minutes to complete. Considering the success of this activity, the 12 individuals who took part in the pre-test were included in the study sample.

1.4.4 Data collection

The data was collected between April and December 2012 by the researcher and another medical student, who had been previously instructed and trained to conduct the interview, during a home visit that had been previously scheduled by telephone or in person, at a time available to the interviewee, at a single point in time. More than one individual could be interviewed in the same household.

1.5 Ethical aspects of research

After authorisation from the Municipal Health Department (**Annex B**), the project was submitted to the Research Ethics Committee of the University of Franca - UNIFRAN, which approved it on 16/12/2011, under number 0087/11 (**Annex C**).

In the Informed Consent Form (**Appendix A**), the ethical principles of beneficence and non-maleficence were taken into account, as well as the participant's right to anonymity, their autonomy to refuse to take part in the research at any time, without prejudice to the follow-up and treatment of the disease, according to Resolution No. 196/96 of the National Research Ethics Council[69] .

Before the interview, each participant was briefed on the objectives of the study, the importance of their participation, clarification of the ICF, the risks and benefits related to the research, the secrecy and confidentiality of the information and the guarantee that there would be no expense, compensation and/or indemnity for this. After agreeing to take part in the study, they signed two copies, one in their possession and the other with the researcher.

1.6 Data analyses

The data collected was stored in a specific database for this study in the EPI INFO computer programme version 3.3.5. The data was descriptively analysed using frequencies, means, medians and percentages. The answers to the open questions were recorded in full and presented in such a way as to enable each participant's view of the content covered.

CHAPTER 4

RESULTS

Based on the objective proposed by the study, the data collected was presented according to the sequence of the data collection instrument, namely: identification data, human biology data, environmental data, lifestyle data and data on the organisation of health services.

4.1 Identification data

Analysing the data obtained from the 40 hypertensive patients who met the inclusion criteria, **Table 1** shows that 23 (57.5%) were female and 17 (42.5%) male. The average age was 47.9 (± 9.8) and the median was 51 years. The most common age group was 51 to 60 years (55.0%), followed by 29 to 40 years (25.0%).

Of the total sample, the majority were married (65.0%) and divorced (20.0%). The average number of children was 2.4 (±1.3).

Table 1: Distribution of hypertensive individuals registered with the Community Health Agent Programme in a municipality in Minas Gerais (2011), according to sex, age group and marital status.

Features	Frequency	
	N°	%
Sex		
Female	23	57,5
Male	17	42,5
Total	40	100
Age group		
51 - 60	22	55,0
29 - 40	10	25,0
41 - 50	7	17,5
18 - 28	1	2,5
Total	40	100
Marital status		
Married	26	65,0
Divorced/separated	8	20,0
Single	4	10,0
Friend	1	2,5
Widowed	1	2,5
Total	40	100

4.2 Human biology data

Of the 40 participants, the most common colour was white, 32 (80.0%), followed by black, 4 (10.0%). The average number of years since medical diagnosis of hypertension was 7.4 (± 7) years. Of all the participants, 38 (95.0%) had been using antihypertensive medication for an average of 4.4 (± 4.3) years.

With regard to adherence to drug treatment, 34 (85.0%) reported that even when they felt well or when their BP was close to values considered normal, they took their antihypertensives. Of the 6 (15.0%) who didn't take their medication every day, 3 (50.0%) claimed it was because they forgot, to assess whether their pressure would rise and one reported that when he went to drink beer, he didn't take his medication. The average number of days for the two interviewees who reported how many days they went without their medication was 5 (± 2.8) days.

When asked about their BP values, according to their last measurement before the interview, in their usual environment (home, health centre, pharmacy), 22 (55.0%) reported BP levels < 140/90mmHg. The rest reported BP levels > 140/90 mmHg.

The antihypertensive drugs most commonly reported by the interviewees were Hydrochlorothiazide (52.5%), Losartan (27.5%), Captopril (20.0%), Enalapril maleate (17.5%), Atenolol (15.0%) and Propranolol hydrochloride (12.5%). Participants could refer to more than one antihypertensive drug, depending on the type of treatment for hypertension. The majority of individuals, 23 (57.5%), were treated with a combination of two, three or four drugs, 15 (37.5%) were treated with monotherapy and 2 (5.0%) did not use any antihypertensive drugs. Of those interviewed, 8 (20.%) reported using simvastatin.

Table 2 shows the risk factors for hypertension and its complications. It can be seen that cardiovascular family history was the most frequently cited by 34 (85.0%) of the participants who reported having at least one first-degree relative with some pathology associated with SAH.

Among the other most cited risk factors were overweight/obesity, 21 (52.5%), and a sedentary lifestyle, 17 (42.5%). Among the complications resulting from AH, the most cited were tachycardia, 5 (12.5%), and AMI, 2 (5.0%). It is worth bearing in mind that the same participant could mention more than one risk factor or complication resulting from AH.

Table 2- Distribution of hypertensive individuals registered with the Community Health Agent Programme in a municipality in Minas Gerais (2011), according to risk factors for SAH and complications resulting from the disease.

Risk factors*	N°	%
Family history cardiovascular	34	85,0
Overweight/Obesity	21	52,5
Sedentary lifestyle	17	42,5
Dyslipidaemia	15	37,5
Diabetes Mellitus	5	12,5
Smoking	3	7,5
Complications arising from AH*		
Tachycardia	5	12,5
Acute Myocardial Infarction	2	5,0
Depression	2	2,5
Angina	1	2,5

*Multiple answers possible.

4.3 Environmental data

The main socio-economic characteristics of the sample are shown in **Table 3**. In terms of level of education, 18 (45.0%) individuals had completed and incomplete primary and secondary education, respectively, and 4 (10.0%) had completed higher education. The majority of participants had a family income of two to three minimum wages, 20 (50.0%), and three to six, 13 (32.5%). The average number of people who depended on this income was 3.4 (± 1.9). As for the participants' work situation, the majority were working - 23 (57.5%). The average working time was 13 (± 12.9) years and the average weekly working day was 45.9 (± 12.4) hours. The average time since retirement and leave of absence was 6.5 (± 5.9) years.

Table 3- Distribution of hypertensive individuals registered with the Community Health Agent Programme in a municipality in Minas Gerais (2011), according to level of education, family income and work situation.

	N°	%
Level of education		
First degree complete/ incomplete	18	45,0
High school complete/ incomplete	18	45,0
Complete university degree	4	10,0
Total	40	100
Income		
2 a 3	20	50,0
3 a 6	13	32,5
6 a 10	4	10,0
Ate 1	3	7,5
Total	40	100
Work situation		
Active	23	57,5
Home	7	17,5
Retired	6	15,0
Away	3	7,5
Unemployed	1	2,5
Total	40	100

4.4 Lifestyle data

With regard to eating habits, 33 (82.5%) said they used sodium restrictions and 7 (17.5%) did not, but both groups were unable to say how many grams of sodium they consumed a day. Among the participants who were on a low-sodium diet, of the 32 who answered the question about who had given them advice, 14 (43.8%) said it was the PACS doctor and among the 14 who said it wasn't the doctor who had given them advice, 11 (78.6%) said it was an acquaintance or family member.

With regard to the consumption of alcoholic drinks, 24 (60.0%) participants reported not using any alcoholic drinks. Of the 16 (40.0%) who did, 9 (56.3%) were male. Beer was mentioned by 14 (82.4%) of the interviewees and the average daily consumption was 4.6 (± 2.5) cans.

Of the 39 interviewees who answered the question about smoking, 9 (23.1%) reported being ex-smokers, 4 (10.3%) reported having used cigarettes for an average of 36.6 years, but were not willing to mention the number of cigarettes/day.

The practice of physical exercise was reported by 23 (57.5%) individuals who said they practised physical activity, with an average duration of 59.5 (± 10.3) minutes and an average in years of 6 (± 11.3) years, with walking being the activity most cited by the interviewees. Of these, 10 (43.5%) reported doing it three times a week and 5 (21.7%) twice a week. Of the 17 (42.5%) who classified themselves as sedentary, the majority claimed lack of time (37.5%), discouragement (25.0%) and body pain (18.8%) as reasons for not doing it.

Of the participants, 25 (62.5%) reported changes in their habits and lifestyle to control BP, with salt and alcohol reduction being the most frequently cited.

Table 4 shows the frequencies and percentages of the places where the interviewees reported monitoring their blood pressure. The majority, 18 (45.0%), said that it was measured at the pharmacy and 12 (30.0%) at the health unit - PACS. Of the 38 interviewees who answered about the frequency of BP measurement, the majority, 15 (39.5%), reported that it was monthly.

Table 4 - Distribution of hypertensive individuals registered with the Community Health Agent Programme in a municipality in Minas Gerais (2011), according to blood pressure monitoring location and frequency.

Location	N°	%
Pharmacy	18	45,0
PACS	12	30,0
At home	7	17,5
Others	2	5,0
Neighbour	1	2,5
Total	40	100
Frequency		
Monthly	15	39,5
Weekly	8	21,1
Almost never	7	18,4
3 times/week	4	10,5
Half-yearly	3	7,9
Daily	1	2,6
Total	38	100

4.5 Data related to the organisation of health services.

When analysing the data related to the organisation of health services, it was noted that 9 (22.5%) said they had private health insurance, even though they used the public service. The rest (77.5%) said they only used public health services to treat their hypertension. When asked which health service they learnt about their diagnosis, the majority, 34 (85.0%), said that they had used a public health service and 6 (15.0%) said that they had used a private health service.

When asked if they followed up with the PACS doctor to treat their hypertension, 37 (92.5%) said yes, 2 (5.0%) said they didn't and 1 (2.5%) mentioned that they were followed up by the health insurance company. Of the 34 who answered about the frequency of these consultations, 17 (50.0%) reported twice a year, 15 (44.1%) once a year, 2 (5.9%) three times a year and six were not willing to answer.

When asked about the initial medical treatment after the diagnosis of hypertension, 27 (67.5%) replied that drug treatment was started immediately, 4 (10.0%) that they were advised and encouraged to adopt changes in their habits and lifestyle and 9 (22.5%) mentioned both.

With regard to access to medical prescriptions for antihypertensive drugs, of the 39 who reported this, 27 (69.2%) said that they went to the health centre to pick them up, 8 (20.5%) said that the health worker took the prescription to their home and 4 (10.3%) said that a family member picked up the prescription at the health centre. With regard to the supply of antihypertensive medication, 39 (97.5%) said they got their medication from the Municipal Pharmacy and one from a private pharmacy.

With regard to the existence of meetings, lectures or discussion groups on SAH in the PACS health units in 2011, 22 (55.0%) said yes, and the majority reported that they were held annually and that the unit's nurse was the one who gave them.

Considering the relevance of the interviewees' participation in these meetings for clarification and guidance on healthy lifestyle habits related to SAH, some participants expressed the following opinions regarding their importance:

> [...] they told me to do physical activity, watch my diet and take my blood pressure (Subject 3).

> [...] I think more about my life, I learn to take more care of myself, my children (Subject 17).

> It didn't add any knowledge, but it did measure the pressure (Subject 10).

> [...] we talked about the things that need to be done for the medicine to work, reducing the salt (Subject32).

With regard to attendance at scheduled activities, 18 (56.3 per cent) of the 32 respondents said they did not take part, the main reasons being lack of time and incompatible working hours.

Table 5 shows the frequency of CHW visits to the interviewees' homes. Of the 39 respondents, 18 (46.2%) reported one visit per month. The same proportion of respondents reported a visit every 45 days and a visit every 90 days (17.9%). When asked about the possibility of replacing their health worker when they were on holiday or on sick leave, 30 (75.0%) reported that there was no replacement, meaning that they were left without the assistance of the CHW at home.

Table 5 - Distribution of hypertensive individuals registered with the Community Health Agent Programme in a municipality in Minas Gerais (2011), according to the frequency of visits by the health agent to their homes.

	N°	%
Frequency of visit		
One visit/month	18	46,2
One visit /45 days	7	17,9
One visit /90 days	7	17,9
One visit /2 months	6	15,4
Half-yearly	1	2,6
Total	39	100

The majority, 21 (52.5%), said that in 2011 they were accompanied by the same team of doctor, nurse and health worker. Among the 19 (47.5%) who reported changes in the health unit's professional staff, the doctor was mentioned by the majority, 10 (52.7%) of those interviewed, followed by the nurse, 4 (21.0%).

Of the total sample, 35 (87.5 per cent) participants reported that they did not encounter any difficulties in monitoring and treating SAH. The main difficulties reported by the participants can be seen in the following statements:

> [...] the difficulty is when you need the tests, and they're not available. Or they don't make the requests (Subject 37).

> [...] the difficulty is on my part, because I forget to go to meetings (Subject17).

> [...] it's difficult to get an appointment. It takes a long time. You have to insist to get an appointment with the doctor (Subject 12).

> The difficulty is getting a doctor, making an appointment isn't difficult [...] (Subject 16).

With regard to knowledge about SAH and its implications, 7 (17.5%) reported having some doubts about the disease, which are represented in the following statements:

> There are people whose hypertension gives them a heart attack? (Subject 40).
> Does it come from the person's genetics? (Subject 32).

> I have a good idea about the subject, but I may be missing something [...] (Subject 8).

> We think we know. We don't really know (Subject 17).

> When there is, I go online (Subject 18).

> Can hypertensive patients do physical activity? So, start walking
> alone? How often? I'm afraid of doing something wrong [...] (Subject 24).

When it came to evaluating the care and follow-up provided by health professionals at the health centre (**Table 6**), 20 (50.0%) reported good care and 11 (27.5%) regular care.

Table 6 - Distribution of hypertensive individuals registered with the Community Health Agent Programme in a municipality in Minas Gerais (2011), according to their assessment of care and follow-up by health professionals.

Evaluation of care and follow-up		
	N°	**%**
Good	20	50,0
Regular	11	27,5
Great	6	15,0
Bad	3	7,5
Total	40	100

When asked if they felt limited by being hypertensive, 10 (25.0%) reported positively. The main limitations reported by the interviewees are represented in the following statements:

> At king's festivals I suffer, but I eat (Subject 13).
> Having to reduce salt and not being able to drink (Subject 17).

> [...] having to worry all the time (Subject 14).

I feel limited at parties [...] (Subject 6).

For me, the difficulty is getting the salt out [...] (Subject 13).

4.6   Analysis of responses related to the organisation of health services.

In order to give more context to the data related to the open questions on the organisation of health services, Table 1 was drawn up with some illustrative statements:

About the health service where you were registered and monitored	*I have nothing to complain about. it's just that I don't go after things [...] (Subject 22).* *n boer mar nfando nou láeo médico não esíá nuem faz rece/to é a enfrrmeiaa e se na farmáciã menicinãO não ter as aemedins, aa faemáciã aaeticunãr eles não accept a receita, por não ter o CRM (Subject 39).* *dolta doctor posted them to us, but the tests haven't been read yet (Subject 20).* *There's no follow-up, you just exchange prescriptions without the doctor seeing you (Subject 23).* *[...m emnona ficarnu muitn tempn without a doctor, I was always attended to (Subject 34).* *The service is satisfactory and I still have health insurance [...] (Subject 27).* *For me, who doesn't have many illnesses, it's fine, but for others it needs to improve [...] (Subject 25).*
What would you like to see changed in the care provided?	*29r a doctor on the days he needs to, because 2)ness doesn't set a day or a time (Subject 29).* *The cleanliness of the post should be better, especially the drinking fountains...] (Subject 6).* *It's difficult to say because I don't go there very often [...] (Subject 21).* *I don't know, I don't have those demands, no (Subject 32).* *Make the recipe last longer [...] (Subject 14).* *[...] that the government should invest more there (Subject 31).* *m...] m doctor [mecira mvir, m <mtavr mom chest pain and he referred me to the neurologist (Subject 16).* *Attention. I'd like a doctor who knows me and a health worker to come to my house...] (Subject 20).* *They've asked for tests, but they don't do them and they suggest going private [...] (Subject 25).* *If medical appointments were already booked, even a year in advance, it would give us more of an obligation to go (Subject 3).* *I don't know. Ah, there's nothing, right? (Subject 5).*
How did you feel about the care and follow-up	*[...] doctors are very uneducated, they think because it's public, it's free, they can be*

provided by health professionals - doctors, nurses and CHAs?	*like that [...] (Subject 10).* *I think it's good with the new agent, because the old one didn't explain anything, the new one does [...] (Subject 17).* *Everyone is good: the doctor, the nurse and the agent (Subjectol).*
	The doctor is a horse, he won't let you talk f...] (Subject 6). *They are attentive and explain everything (Subject 36).* *The nurses and health workers are great, except for the doctor (Subject 9).* *Sometimes it's not the whole team's fault, but it leaves something to be desired [...] (Subject 11).*
Space reserved for comments	*If the neighbourhood offered a place to go to the gym later in the day it would be good, there's no incentive [...] (Subject 16).* *When there's no medicine in the municipal pharmacy and I go to buy the medicine in normal pharmacies, the prescription isn't valid because it doesn't have the CRM. That's bad, isn't it? (Subject 39).* *The only thing I don't think is right is that doctors change a lot. He does an examination with one and shows it to another (Subject 20).* *Now, the staff there are all the most attentive, because at the other post, it wasn't like that (Subject 36).* *[...] and what about my case? I need test requests, RNI every fortnight and the appointment with the doctor is once a year (Subject 33).* *[...] they need to humanise the staff, because the people who go there are already suffering[...]* *[..]* *I remember that song "ah, cattle life, marked people, happy people" (Subject 12).* *The doctors are good and so are the nurses, but I don't see the staff (Subject 29).* *[...] the times I went there, I thought it was great (Subject 7).*

Chart 1: Distribution of the opinions of hypertensive individuals registered with the municipality's Community Health Agent Programme (2011), in relation to certain questions.

CHAPTER 5

DISCUSSION

Based on the study's aim of describing the living and health conditions of hypertensive individuals registered and monitored by the Community Health Agents Programme (PACS) in a municipality in Minas Gerais, from the perspective of the four elements of the Health Field model, the discussion will be described and presented in the same sequence as the data collection instrument and the results.

5.1 Identification data

The results of this study showed that 23 (57.5%) of the participants were female. Data related to the higher occurrence of hypertension in women has also been found in national studies[17, 18, 70-73]. The higher prevalence of hypertensive women compared to men may be related to women's greater demand for health services, demonstrating a probable concern for their health. Women generally take on the task of providing medical care for the family, and are more present in health services, making it possible to diagnose problems[9, 74].

A study carried out in Bambuí - MG([17]), whose main objective was to determine the prevalence of AH in the municipality, showed a prevalence of 44.9%, with 26.9% for females and 22.0% for males.

A divergent result was found in a study in São Paulo - SP, which pointed to a higher prevalence of hypertension in men. The aim of the study was to find out the prevalence of hypertension in 864 employees of a hospital complex and relate it to socio-demographic variables. The prevalence of SAH was found to be higher in males, in individuals aged 50 or over[75].

The prevalent age range in this study was 51 to 60 years (55.0%). The mean age was 47.9 ($\pm$ 9.8) years, median 51 years, with a minimum age of 24 and a maximum age of 60.

In Brazil, the diagnosis of SAH becomes more prevalent with age, reaching around 5.0 per cent of individuals aged between 18 and 24 and more than 50.0 per cent in the 65 and over age group[71].

A study carried out in Umuarama - PR, which aimed to describe adherence to non-pharmacological antihypertensive treatment among users of a School Health Centre, pointed to a higher prevalence in the 51 to 60 age group (31.9%), corroborating the data found in this study[76]. It is known that BP and the severity of its elevation increase with age. This can be explained by the physical changes that come with ageing, such as loss of arterial compliance, which makes the individual more prone to developing hypertension, as well as by the psychological and social changes that affect individuals with prolonged life spans[2, 9, 72].

Population ageing in Brazil has led to a new profile of users of health services, pointing to the need to plan care for people with chronic diseases such as SAH. The actions to be planned should be geared towards the specific needs of this population and should prioritise the monitoring of health conditions, with preventive and differentiated health and education actions, with qualified care and multidimensional and comprehensive care[77].

The greater occurrence of married people (65.0%) and divorced people (20.0%) in the study can be explained by the fact that the prevalent age group in the sample was concentrated among individuals aged over 29 (97.5%).

The higher number of married individuals corroborates the study that aimed to estimate the prevalence of hypertension in the population and identify the sociodemographic factors of hypertensive patients[9]. The result found was 63.9% of married hypertensive patients, justifying that, possibly, the higher prevalence of hypertension in married individuals could have been due to the degree of family responsibility, which could be a risk factor for hypertension.

On the other hand, marital status has been shown to facilitate adherence to treatment, i.e. having a partner can promote the process of treating SAH[78].

5.2 Human biology data

The human biology element, which in the Health Field model includes all the factors related to health, both physical and mental, that manifest themselves in the body as a consequence of the fundamental biology and organic constitution of the individual, relates to the person's genetic inheritance, the maturing and ageing process and the different systems, organs and internal apparatus of the human body. This element contributes to all types of illness and mortality, including chronic communicable and non-communicable diseases[1].

Considering the possible changes in the body caused by hypertension, the data contained in the form was analysed in order to help identify the presence of risk factors and the complications caused by hypertension.

The prevalence of SAH in non-white individuals is described in the literature as being almost twice as high as in white individuals, with the genetic hypothesis being responsible for this fact[2, 9].

The most common colour in this study was white, with 80.0%. This result corroborates other studies[9, 71] which found prevalences of 78.4% and 84.0%, respectively. It differs from a study carried out in Recife - PE, with patients in hypertensive crisis between May 2001 and October 2002, which showed that 75% of the patients seen during this period were classified as non-white[79].

The average number of years since medical diagnosis of hypertension in this study was 7.4 (± 7) years and 6.8 (± 7.3) years since treatment. Over the years following a diagnosis of hypertension, individuals can become accustomed to this pathological condition, and what was initially new and could be feared becomes routine. The individual stops taking the necessary precautions and positions themselves as a manipulator of the disease. The various everyday situations lead the individual to challenge the disease and analyse its outcome[76].

Drug treatment with antihypertensives was reported by 95.0% of the participants and with regard to adherence, 85.0% reported taking their medication daily, although 45.0% of the interviewees mentioned BP levels > 140/90 mmHg, i.e. they did not have controlled BP levels. The interviewees (15.0%) who didn't take their medication every day claimed that they forgot, that they were trying to assess the effectiveness of the treatment, i.e. whether their BP would rise without the medication, and when they were going to drink alcohol.

These results are similar to a study carried out in Minas Gerais[16] , which aimed to estimate the prevalence of SAH and identify associated socioeconomic, demographic and anthropometric variables. The results showed that 54.5% of the individuals who reported taking their medication at the right times and in the right doses had high BP levels.

A study carried out in Rio Grande de Sul[80] , which aimed to describe the prevalence of SAH risk factors in the state's adult population, the level of recognition and control of the disease, as well as associated factors, found that 30.1% of individuals reported following antihypertensive treatment, but did not have adequate BP control. In view of this result, the authors consider that it is clear that adherence and effective control of SAH have not yet reached a satisfactory level, representing a challenge to be faced by the health system.

In a study carried out in São Luís-MA, which sought to identify the drugs most used by hypertensive patients and their associations, their blood pressure levels and to estimate adherence to treatment, 75% reported adhering to drug treatment and those who did not follow reported forgetfulness, the feeling of not needing to use the medication and the side effects caused by the medication as justifications[81] .

Adherence has been the word widely used in the health field to characterise when medical or health advice coincides with the individual's behaviour, in terms of taking prescribed medication, making lifestyle changes and attending medical appointments[71, 82] . It is a complex behavioural process that is greatly influenced by the environment, the health system and health care[78] .

Long-term adherence to treatment for chronic diseases such as hypertension is low. It is around 50 per cent in developed countries and 20 per cent in developing countries. Although patients are blamed for not following the prescribed regimens, non-adherence is fundamentally a failure of the health system[83] .

The main reasons for non-adherence to antihypertensive treatment are: the patient's lack of knowledge about the disease or motivation to treat an asymptomatic but chronic disease, low socioeconomic status, cultural aspects and mistaken beliefs acquired from experiences with the disease in the family context, inadequate relationship with the health team and prolonged time between appointments due to scheduling difficulties, medication side effects and interference with quality of life after starting treatment[19, 54] .

Increasing adherence to antihypertensive drug treatment and especially non-drug treatment is the responsibility of the multi-professional team, through health education, with a special focus on concepts about hypertension and its long-term consequences, understandable and detailed guidance on medication and its side effects and, above all, the benefits of lifestyle changes[2, 28]

SAH is one of the main causes of hospitalisation in the SUS and is related to the development of other chronic diseases and complications. Given this magnitude, the Ministry of Health has adopted various strategies and actions to reduce this burden on the Brazilian population, including the free distribution of medicines[84] .

In 2004, the Popular Pharmacy Programme of Brazil was created, a partnership between the three spheres of government, with the aim of increasing the population's access to medicines considered essential, passing them on at a low cost. This strategy was extended to the private network of pharmacies and drugstores in 2006, receiving the name Aqui Tem Farmácia Popular. Under this programme, the Ministry of Health subsidised 90% of the reference value of the 24 medicines available for AH, DM, asthma, rhinitis, Parkinson's disease, osteoporosis and glaucoma[84] .

In March 2011, the Saúde Não Tem Preço (Health is Priceless) programme was created with the aim of increasing access to medicines for hypertensive and diabetic individuals. Pharmacies and drugstores affiliated with the Aqui Tem Farmácia Popular network now offer 11 free medicines for the treatment of these diseases. The antihypertensive drugs provided for the treatment of hypertension are: Hydrochlorothiazide, Losartan, Captopril, Enalapril maleate, Atenolol and Propranolol hydrochloride[84] .

In this study, the antihypertensive drugs most often reported by the interviewees were part of the medicines provided by the Saúde Não Tem Preço Programme, such as hydrochlorothiazide (52.5%), losartan (27.5%), captopril (20.0%), enalapril maleate (17.5%), atenolol (15.0%) and propranolol hydrochloride (12.5%).

The majority of individuals (57.5%) were treated with a combination of two, three or four drugs, 37.5% were treated with monotherapy and 5.0% did not use any antihypertensive drugs.

This result corroborates a study carried out in Fortaleza-CE[85] which aimed to investigate the behavioural aspects of following pharmacological and non-pharmacological therapy and the degree of adherence to antihypertensive treatment in a specific group. The results showed that 26 (53.0%) were taking combined therapy and 23 (47.0%) monotherapy.

These results do not corroborate the study carried out in São Luíz-MA, which found that 66.0% of interviewees cited monotherapy as the antihypertensive therapeutic regimen most often prescribed by doctors[81] .

An important fact to note is that 20.0% of those interviewed reported using simvastatin, a drug used to treat dyslipidaemia, to reduce levels of bad cholesterol (LDL) and triglycerides, increasing levels of good cholesterol (HDL) in the blood and reducing the risk of CVD[86] . This result was to be expected given that most hypertensive patients have risk factors associated with hypertension such as being overweight or obese, dyslipidaemia and a sedentary lifestyle. In this study, 37.5% of the interviewees reported having high cholesterol.

Given this reality, the importance of trained health teams to provide adequate guidance on the correct use of medicines, the action and expected result of each one and the importance of individual adherence to drug and non-drug treatments stands out[5, 19].

Considering the reduction of BP levels in hypertension as the sole objective of anti-hypertensive therapy is not the most appropriate because, in addition to being a multifactorial disease, it depends on the collaboration and active participation of the hypertensive individual for its treatment and control. When not properly treated, hypertension can have serious consequences for the individual, and is one of the most frequent causes of morbidity and mortality in adults and the elderly, making it a major challenge for health professionals[17, 87].

Risk factors such as older age, obesity, family history of AH, level of education and alcohol abuse are significantly associated with the prevalence of SAH[88], i.e. the prevalence of the disease increases as risk factors are added[17].

With regard to cardiovascular family history, 34 (85.0%) of the interviewees reported a family history of SAH, showing that heredity is a risk factor for its onset. This is in line with the results of other studies[89-91] which found 70.0%, 70.0% and 50.8%, respectively, of participants who reported a cardiovascular family history.

The worldwide epidemic of overweight, whether overweight or obese, was also evident in this study, with 52.5%, as in other studies[70, 72]. The strong association between excess weight and the occurrence of AH is almost linear and indicates the urgency of measures capable of acting on the risk factors that can decisively interfere in determining the prevalence of AH[29, 70]. For every 10kg of weight reduced, there is an approximate reduction in SBP of 5 to 20 mmHg, i.e. loss of body weight is associated with reductions in BP in overweight people. In addition to excess weight, low frequency of physical activity also contributes to the increased prevalence of AH[29].

Obesity in middle-aged adults has reached alarming proportions, which is partly related to the lack of physical activity and the modern lifestyle in which most free time is spent on sedentary activities such as watching television, using computers and driving around[92].

Obesity, hypertension and DM should be managed clinically as a chronic condition, and treatment should be focussed on a lifelong approach. When an individual is overweight or obese, the medical history and clinical examination should be centred on the causes and complications of obesity. Once the risk associated with it has been established, the motivation for weight loss should be addressed[93].

AH and DM are frequently associated clinical conditions. The possibility of this association is as high as 50 per cent, which requires the management of both conditions in the same patient[92]. They share some aspects and risk factors, such as obesity, dyslipidaemia, sedentary lifestyle, non-drug treatment, the need to change lifestyle habits, ease of diagnosis and difficult adherence, and should be monitored by a multidisciplinary team, among others[28, 92].

Considering the high risk of cardiovascular events, it is important and recommended that diabetic individuals maintain blood pressure levels of up to 130/80 mmHg. In order to achieve the proposed target, the indicated therapy should include, in addition to the appropriate use of drugs, weight reduction, physical exercise, moderation in salt and alcohol consumption and quitting smoking[93].

In this study, 12.5% of the interviewees reported being diabetic and 42.5% sedentary. Of these, most claimed lack of time and discouragement as reasons for not practising physical activity. A similar result was described in a study in Fortaleza - CE, which aimed to describe the non-pharmacological treatment followed by a group of elderly hypertensive patients, in an attempt to subsidise nursing care. Approximately 35.0% of those interviewed reported being sedentary and all of them had some failure to adhere to the antihypertensive therapy instituted[87]. In a study carried out in the municipality of Ribeirão Preto - SP, in a basic health unit, with diabetic and hypertensive users, 63.3% reported being sedentary.[72]

National estimates point to a high level of sedentary lifestyles in our population, with more than half of people doing little or no physical activity[92]. A sedentary lifestyle is one of the most important risk factors for the development of NCDs, including hypertension, together with an inadequate diet and smoking. It is related to a high prevalence of hypertension and leads to diseases that represent a significant economic cost, both for individuals and for society, due to the sequelae they cause[88, 92, 94].

Increasing the population's knowledge and involvement in the benefits of physical activity is an important strategy for controlling and preventing hypertension. The aim is to get sedentary people to become active, incorporating physical activity into their life routine[92].

Complications resulting from AH were reported by 25.0% of the participants, including tachycardia, AMI, depression and angina.

In the descriptive and retrospective study, which aimed to characterise the profile of hypertensive users registered and monitored by a Family Health Unit in a municipality in the interior of eastern Minas Gerais, among the complications related to AH from the Hiperdia form, kidney disease and AMI stood out among hypertensive users[95].

AH is responsible for cardiovascular, cerebral, coronary, renal and peripheral vascular complications. It is estimated that 40% of strokes and 25% of AMIs in hypertensive patients could be prevented with adequate antihypertensive therapy[33]. In the heart, the characteristic lesion of AH is hypertrophy of the left ventricle, with an increase in weight and a decrease in the cavity. This increase in left ventricular mass is not accompanied by an increase in coronary circulation, which causes a change between energy expenditure and supply, leading to myocardial ischaemia and, consequently, angina and tachycardia.[92]

Depression is a complication of hypertension that is rarely mentioned. It is important to emphasise the lack of awareness of the disease among the population and also people's fear of talking about the problem[71].

5.3 Environmental data

This category includes all health-related aspects external to the human body, belonging to the physical or social environments and over which the individual has little or no control (control of air and water and control of social changes and their effects on health)[1].

The assessment of socioeconomic status is based on the type of occupation and level of education, with higher rates of SAH being observed in lower socioeconomic levels. Socioeconomic differences play an important role in health conditions as a result of various factors, such as access to the health system, level of information, understanding of the problem and adherence to treatment[9, 16].

When we looked at the level of education of the study participants, we found the same proportion (45.0%) of individuals with complete and incomplete primary and secondary education. Some Brazilian studies have found an association between hypertension and educational level[75, 88]. In the study carried out in São José do Rio Preto[9], SAH was more prevalent among individuals with less schooling in all age groups.

In Brazil, individuals with up to eight years of schooling are the ones who most often report a medical diagnosis of AH. Among women, there is an association between level of schooling and diagnosis of the disease, because while 32.8 per cent with up to eight years of schooling report a diagnosis of hypertension, the same condition is observed in 13.6 per cent of women with 12 or more years of schooling[71].

The level of education plays an important role in the planning and implementation of educational activities. The information should be in easy-to-understand language, facilitating communication and aimed at the understanding and participation of individuals with AH in the proposed guidelines[2, 71, 72].

Low levels of education can hinder access to information and understanding of the complex mechanisms of the disease and treatment, restricting learning opportunities related to health care, such as understanding diet, prescribed medication and the importance of physical activity. Schooling is a variable to be taken into account when designing an educational programme for this clientele[72].

With regard to occupation, 57.5% of the participants were active. Studies on the prevalence of SAH[71, 96] consider that the occupation of individuals and the characteristics of their work, including lack of autonomy, work under severe supervision, job instability and job dissatisfaction, can raise BP.

A study carried out in the São Paulo metropolitan region on the prevalence of hypertension showed that women in the labour market had no risk factors for hypertension. On the other hand, those who did not work and had a sedentary lifestyle had an increased rate of obesity and BP. These findings show that people who keep active can achieve personal satisfaction, greater social interaction, improved mental and physical health, contributing to a reduction in stress and depression and, consequently, a better quality of life[97].

Most of the participants (82.5 per cent) had a family income of between two and six minimum wages. The average number of people who depended on this income was 3.4 (+ 1.9).

This result is similar to a study carried out at an endocrinology outpatient clinic in a health centre in the city of São Paulo, which aimed to characterise hypertensive patients and find out about their main difficulties in adhering to the treatment proposed by the health team. The results showed that 63.0% had a monthly family income of between two and five or more minimum wages[98] .

The influence of the socio-economic profile, represented by low income and low schooling, on BP control plays an important role in health conditions as a result of various factors, such as access to the health system, the degree of information and understanding of the problem, adherence to treatment, indicating that people with less favoured socio-economic conditions have higher blood pressure levels[9, 75, 89] .

Low socioeconomic status is identified as a limiting factor for effective BP control, but this relationship has been questioned, thus indicating the need to broaden the concepts inherent in the relationship between social and economic factors and the health-disease process[78, 99] . Socioeconomic status alone may not be solely responsible for low adherence to treatment and consequent unsatisfactory control of the disease, but it is an important social marker and its action will undoubtedly reflect on the problem of the disease and treatment .[78]

5.4 Lifestyle data

Lifestyle data make up a set of individual decisions that affect health and over which it is possible to exercise a certain degree of control. For health, lifestyle, through choices, personal habits, correct or incorrect decisions, determines the actions that will directly influence the individual's level of health[1] .

Several authors have pointed out that NCDs, including hypertension, result from the interaction of genetic, environmental and lifestyle factors. The most investigated aspects of lifestyle that constitute risk factors for hypertension are high-sodium diets, sedentary lifestyles, obesity and excessive alcohol consumption. Modifying these risk factors can prevent or delay the onset of hypertension or even delay the complications resulting from the disease, favouring an improved quality of life and reducing costs for the health system[5, 29, 83] .

In view of the interest in knowing the influence of this element on the occurrence of SAH in the population under study, some data related to eating habits, smoking and physical activity were sought.

Diet is considered one of the most important modifiable factors for the prevention and treatment of NCDs, including hypertension, and should be included among the priority public health actions. An inadequate diet, rich in fats, sodium, highly refined and processed foods and low in fruit and vegetables, is associated with the onset of various diseases such as dyslipidaemias, AH, AMI, DM and cancer[12] .

Changes in eating habits are difficult to incorporate into the routine and must be acquired slowly, gradually. This is due to the fact that eating habits are related to socioeconomic, cultural and social factors[5, 29] .

When trying to investigate the daily consumption of sodium in the diet, the majority (82.5%) reported that they restricted sodium and none of the participants were able to say how much they consumed a day. The amount of sodium recommended in the literature is 5g of sodium chloride or table salt/day, i.e. 2.0g of sodium/day, which corresponds to approximately four teaspoons of salt added to food[5, 29, 87] .

A similar result was described in a study carried out in Fortaleza-CE, where approximately 26% of hypertensive patients reported not controlling their daily salt intake. The study also pointed out that although the majority reported an adequate salt intake, this index was subjective, as there was no way of proving the amount of sodium they ingested on a daily basis[87] .

A meta-analysis carried out in 2003, which evaluated the dose-response between salt reduction and a drop in BP, showed that the reduction in BP is directly proportional to the reduction in the daily amount of salt in the diet. The authors found that a 3g reduction in salt intake in hypertensive patients reduced SBP by 3.6 to 5.6 mmHg and DBP by 1.9 to 3.2 mmHg[29, 100] . Despite individual differences in sensitivity, even modest reductions in salt intake are generally effective in reducing BP[29] .

Among the participants who were on a low-sodium diet, of the 32 who answered the question about who had given them advice, 14 (43.8 per cent) reported the PACS doctor.

In a study carried out in the interior of the state of São Paulo[101] , with the aim of assessing the behaviour of diabetics and hypertensive patients in relation to the treatment and guidance they receive and whether the care provided in family health units meets the guidelines of the Ministry of Health for the care of these diseases, the guidance received on adopting habits for a healthy life (diet, physical activity, smoking) for 50.0% of the participants was provided by the doctor at the time of the consultation. The main advice received regarding diet, as reported by the patients, was to change eating habits (30.0%), reduce salt intake (23.0%) and weight (12.0%). Of those interviewed, 25.0% reported not having received any advice.

Adherence to non-drug treatment, i.e. that which requires changes in habits and lifestyle, such as the discipline of a low-sodium diet and the routine practice of physical activities, requires a lot of effort and determination on the part of the hypertensive patient and guidance from the professionals who assist them[5, 87] .

Health professionals should advise the consumption of natural seasonings such as parsley, chives and aromatic herbs, which are recommended in place of industrialised condiments such as sausages, preserves, canned and smoked foods and salted snacks, which should be avoided[28, 54] .

Hypertensive individuals, like non-hypertensive individuals, should eat a varied diet with a balanced nutrient content, rich in whole grains, fruit, vegetables, meat and low-fat dairy products. Artificial sweeteners can be used, considering their sodium content. The consumption of fibre in the diet should be encouraged in the form of vegetables, legumes, whole grains and fruit, which provide minerals, vitamins and other essential nutrients for a healthy diet[5, 54] .

The lack of adequate guidance and clarification for hypertensive patients about their real health situation, the causes and consequences of the condition, treatment and, above all, the importance and repercussions of changing lifestyle habits for BP control and reduction, can lead to low adherence to non-drug treatment[87] .

With regard to alcohol consumption, 16 (40.0%) participants reported using alcohol. Of these, 9 (56.3%) were male, and beer was mentioned by 14 (82.4%). The average daily consumption of cans of beer (350 ml/can) was 4.6 ($\pm$ 2.5)/day.

There is an association between alcohol intake and changes in BP depending on the amount ingested[5] . A greater amount of ethanol raises BP and is associated with greater cardiovascular morbidity and mortality [29] .

The amount of ethanol ingested per day should be limited to 30 ml for men and 15 ml for women or underweight individuals. This daily amount of ethanol is equivalent to approximately ($\sim$) two cans of beer/day (350 ml/can), one glass of wine ($\sim$300 ml) or three doses of spirits ($\sim$30 ml/dose), such as whisky, vodka and brandy[5, 30] .

Some studies indicate that moderate alcohol consumption can reduce the risk of death from coronary heart disease. However, consumption above the recommended level is associated with numerous social and health consequences and the harms can outweigh the benefits[12] . The WHO defines moderate alcohol consumption as one dose/day for women and two doses/day for men. Intake of daily doses above this standard for prolonged periods of time is considered harmful to health and can increase BP[12, 102] .

Evidence of a correlation between a small intake of alcohol and a consequent reduction in BP is still fragile and needs to be proven. In hypertensive individuals, alcohol intake reduces BP acutely and depending on the dose, but it rises a few hours after consumption[2, 29] . Excessive ethanol consumption in Brazilian populations is associated with the occurrence of hypertension[2, 5] . There are differences in alcohol consumption by gender, with abusive use being more frequent among men .[12]

Studies show that decreases in SBP of up to 4.1 mmHg and DBP of 2.6 mmHg can occur just by reducing ethanol consumption[5, 29, 30] . The health team should be attentive to the consumption of alcohol by hypertensive patients, because in addition to the direct effect of alcohol on the activation of the sympathetic nervous system, causing an increase in BP, it also affects drug treatment, as the individual does not use the medication to drink alcoholic beverages[5, 30, 87] .

In view of the controversy regarding the safety and cardiovascular benefits of low doses, as well as the harmful effects of alcohol on society, health professionals should advise people who drink alcoholic beverages not to exceed 30g of ethanol/day for men and 15g for women, and that drinking should not become a habit[5, 12] .

With regard to smoking, of the 39 interviewees who answered about their cigarette consumption, 9 (23.1%) said they were ex-smokers and 4 (10.3%) said they had been smoking for an average of 36.6 years, but were unwilling to mention the number of cigarettes/day. After being diagnosed with SAH, 3 (75.0%) of the participants reported reducing their consumption.

A similar result was found in a study carried out in Sacramento-MG[71] , with the aim of characterising individuals with AH who took part in the educational group, where 8.4% of the participants reported an average smoking time of 41 years. The number of former smokers was also higher (37.4%).

Smoking is one of the main causes of premature death and disability and represents a public health problem, not only in developed countries but also in developing countries. Tobacco increases the risk of premature deaths and physical limitations due to its constrictive effect, which causes acute haemodynamic changes and increases the risk of developing ischaemic heart disease, stroke, pulmonary emphysema, cancer, among others, doubling the risk of coronary artery disease[12, 103] . The Brazilian Hypertension Guidelines[2, 5] recommend that people with hypertension stop smoking.

Even though the use of cigarettes observed in the population studied was a minority, it is important to encourage people to give up smoking as an effective measure to reduce the risk of high BP and the onset of cardiovascular diseases, since most of them have other associated risk factors such as being overweight or obese and a sedentary lifestyle, which together can accelerate the development of complications related to hypertension.

57.5% of those interviewed reported practising physical exercise, with an average duration of 59.5 (± 10.3) minutes and an average in years of 6 (± 11.3) years. The majority (78.2%) reported exercising between two and four times a week, with walking being their favourite activity. Among the 17 (42.5%) hypertensive patients who classified themselves as sedentary, the majority claimed lack of time (37.5%), discouragement (25.0%) and body pain (18.8%) as reasons for not doing them.

This result is similar to that of a study carried out at an endocrinology outpatient clinic in a health centre in the city of São Paulo. Of the total number of people interviewed, 22.2% reported difficulties in taking part in physical activity and the main reasons were pain (25.0%), lack of company (16.7%) and lack of time (16.7%)[98] .

It is recommended for all hypertensive patients, including those under drug treatment, to practice aerobic exercise such as walking, swimming, jogging, dancing, three to five times a week, lasting at least 30 minutes a day. Exercise can reduce SBP by up to 4 to 9 mmHg. It has also been emphasised that hypertensive patients in stage three can only start physical activity once their BP has been controlled[5, 29] .

The health benefits of physical activity have been widely documented in numerous reports, including a reduction in the risk of death from CVD, the risk of developing SAH, DM, colon and breast cancer, improved mental health through reduced anxiety, fatigue and depression, healthier bones and joints, better body function and preservation of independence in the elderly, control of body weight and favourable correlations with a reduction in smoking, alcohol and drug abuse[54] .

The effect of mild to moderate physical exercise on resting BP levels is especially important, since individuals with hypertension can reduce the dosage of their antihypertensive medication, or even have their BP controlled, without the adoption of pharmacological measures[104] . The practice of physical activity is an essential therapy in the treatment of hypertension[72] , as it reduces the incidence of hypertension, even in pre-hypertensive individuals .[2]

With regard to changes in habits and lifestyle to control BP, 62.5 per cent said yes, with salt and alcohol reduction being the most frequently cited.

The main objective of non-drug treatment is to reduce cardiovascular morbidity and mortality through lifestyle changes that favour a reduction in blood pressure and is indicated for all hypertensive patients, regardless of age and BP classification[87] . It requires changes that have been proven to reduce BP, in particular reducing body weight, salt intake and alcohol consumption and regular physical exercise .[5]

Lifestyle changes involved in non-drug treatment should be prescribed and encouraged by health professionals to all hypertensive patients, regardless of their blood pressure levels, as they have been shown to prevent or delay the rise in BP in hypertensive patients with borderline values and to reduce values that are already high[105] . This is not an easy task, as it requires behavioural changes in cultural habits acquired over many years of life, showing the importance of continuous actions with hypertensive patients .[87]

With regard to BP monitoring, 18 (45.0%) interviewees reported measuring it at the pharmacy and 12 (30.0%) at the health unit. Of the 38 interviewees who answered about the frequency of BP measurement, the majority, 15 (39.5%), reported that it was monthly.

BP measurement is a simple procedure, easy to perform and should be carried out in all health assessments, by doctors from different specialities and other health professionals, all of whom should be properly trained. Monitoring BP levels is an important aid in monitoring the effectiveness of drug therapy in hypertensive patients and, above all, in preventing cardiovascular events[5] .

5.5 Data related to the organisation of health services

This data encompasses the practice of health team professionals, hospitals, pharmacies, public and community health services, dental services, among others, and refers to the quality, quantity, administration, nature of relationships between people, as well as the resources available for health care. Generally, the organisation of health services is defined as a health care system, at the preventive, curative and recovery levels, and includes the availability, quality and quantity of resources to provide health care[1] .

Of the population interviewed, 77.5% of the participants reported using only public health services to treat their SAH, 22.5% reported having a private health insurance plan and 85.0% reported having learnt about their SAH diagnosis at a public health institution.

A similar result was found in a study aimed at evaluating the performance of a family health team in caring for people with hypertension in a small town in the state of Paraná in 2003, where 91.8% of the interviewees reported using the public health system (SUS), 5% were users of a health insurance plan with full coverage and 6.4% with partial coverage. The use of private health services was mentioned in 17.2% of cases[106] . This data leads us to conclude that even people who have private health insurance make use of public healthcare.

In Brazil, around 75.0% of the population's healthcare is provided through the public SUS network[2] . All forms of care for hypertensive patients can be carried out at all levels of health care; however, in primary care the field of care is directed towards health guidance and monitoring of hypertensive patients .[107]

Health care geared towards the needs of hypertensive patients, from the implementation of the SUS until the end of the 1990s, was considered fragmented and discontinuous, both in terms of clinical aspects and actions to promote health and reduce risk factors. With regard to care for users with hypertension in the public health system, there was a lack of coordination between the various levels of care within the system, as well as difficulties in improving and qualifying health professionals, resulting in a backlog of patients in specialised services[72] .

Aiming to restructure and expand effective, quality care for users affected by AH and DM in the public health services network, the Ministry of Health implemented the Plan to Reorganise Care for AH and DM, with the aim of reducing the morbidity and mortality profile of these diseases, the number of hospital admissions and early retirements. Its general objective was to establish guidelines and targets for the reorganisation of care for AH and DM, by updating professionals in the basic network, guaranteeing diagnosis and linking patients to health units for treatment and follow-up, thus promoting the restructuring and expansion of resolutive and quality care in the SUS[33, 54] .

This plan consisted of five stages: training multipliers to update primary care professionals; an information campaign to detect suspected cases and promote healthy lifestyle habits; diagnostic confirmation and initiation of treatment; registration and linking of hypertensive and diabetic patients to primary care units, implementation of health care protocols and evaluation of the impact of this plan[33, 54] .

When asked if they followed up with the PACS doctor to treat their hypertension, 92.5% said yes. Of the 34 who answered about the frequency of consultations, 94.1 per cent reported once or twice a year, 5.9 per cent three times a year and six were not willing to answer.

In a study carried out in a small town in the state of Paraná[106] , 35.9% did not see a doctor in 2003, 31.4% saw a doctor up to twice a year, and 21.5% three to five times a year. In a study carried out in São Paulo-SP[108] , over a six-month period, 70.0% of patients attended between three and four appointments, 5.0% six and 10.0% two.

Easy access to the health service promotes greater adherence to treatment and is an item that demonstrates its good quality, identified by the ease with which medical appointments can be booked or with other members of the team[101] .

Although it has not yet been studied, one of the possible indirect ways of inferring one of the facets of adherence to the proposed antihypertensive treatment is by observing attendance at scheduled appointments. This simple measure can show access to the health service, the patient's desire to treat their illness and reveal their awareness of having a health problem that requires care[101, 109] .

When asked about the initial medical treatment after the diagnosis of hypertension, 27 (67.5%) hypertensive patients replied that drug treatment was started immediately, 4 (10.0%) that they were advised and encouraged to adopt changes in their habits and lifestyle and 9 (22.5%) mentioned both behaviours.

The study carried out in Cajazeiras-PB[110] aimed to investigate the knowledge of patients with AH about their treatment. The most cited treatment was the combination of drug and non-drug treatment (61.1%), drug treatment alone (27.7%) and non-drug treatment alone (11.1%).

The continued belief that the use of medication is the best choice for the treatment of AH confirms the biomedical model, centred on the treatment of the disease, with no incentive for changes in lifestyle and eating habits[101] .

It is the doctor's role to educate and encourage the patient, informing them about the clinical significance and prognosis of their illness, as well as the possibilities of drug and non-drug treatment[109] .

Non-drug treatment for hypertension consists of strategies aimed at changing lifestyle and, although it is important and necessary, it is still difficult to implement. Lifestyle changes are an attitude that should be encouraged in all hypertensive patients, regardless of BP level, throughout their lives. These changes in lifestyle habits have proven value in reducing blood pressure levels and the risk of cardiovascular events[111] .

Promoting health among hypertensive individuals consists of developing strategies aimed at changing lifestyles, as a form of intervention for the prevention of sequelae and treatment of hypertension. These changes can lead to a reduction in the dosage of antihypertensive drugs or even their suspension, alleviating the adverse effects of pharmacological treatment and reducing costs for hypertensive patients and the health system. However, professional practice can favour drug treatment, resulting in non-adherence to lifestyle changes and compromising BP control[76, 111] .

With regard to access to medical prescriptions for antihypertensive drugs, of the 39 who reported this, 27 (69.2%) said that they went to the health centre to get them, 8 (20.5%) said that the health worker took the prescription to their home and 4 (10.3%) said that a family member took the prescription to the health centre. Medicines were purchased almost exclusively (97.5%) from the Municipal Pharmacy, reflecting the scope and effectiveness of the programme set up by the Ministry of Health.

Free access to antihypertensive medication is an important factor in BP control[16] .

Regarding meetings, lectures or discussion groups on SAH organised by the PACS health units, 56.3% reported not taking part due to lack of time and incompatible working hours.

This result corroborates the study carried out in São Luíz-MA, which also observed the participation of interviewees in educational activities on hypertension at their respective health centres, finding 55.2% who said they had never participated in lectures or discussions on hypertension[81] .

Guidance and clarification work can be carried out in hypertensive groups, in which it is recommended to develop activities that also involve family members, whenever possible. This work can also be aimed at hypertensive individuals who are being monitored by a private doctor[99] .

Group educational activities provide participants with a constant exchange of information, favour the clarification of doubts and ease anxieties about living with similar problems. They can be implemented through an individual or collective approach, with group educational intervention representing a differential in adherence to treatment[82] . These group interventions to promote self-care promote beneficial interaction between members, allowing for a greater understanding of the problem. They also emphasise the importance of proper planning for groups and the training of coordinators, who must combine knowledge with sensitivity to evaluate the results, seeking the effectiveness of the activities carried out[72] . It is important to always consider cultural particularities when developing any planned activity[5] .

According to the Ministry of Health, primary care prioritises the prevention and control of SAH through educational activities to control risk factors such as obesity, sedentary lifestyles, smoking and the prevention of possible complications[3] .

The results relating to the CHWs' monitoring of hypertensive patients at home showed that visits varied from once a month (46.2%), every 45 days and every 90 days (17.9%), to a minimum frequency of every six months. When the agent was away on holiday or on sick leave, 30 (75.0%) reported that there was no replacement and that they were left without assistance at home.

In the study carried out in Matão-SP[101] , with the aim of identifying and analysing the user's opinion of the assistance and care provided by the family health team, 80.0% of the participants said that CHA visits were regular, i.e. at least once a month.

The ACS is a health professional who is part of the PACS and works exclusively within the SUS. Under the supervision of the local manager, the nurse instructor-supervisor, they carry out disease prevention and health promotion activities through home or community-based, individual or collective actions, developed in accordance with the guidelines incorporated by this system[47, 112] . Among their duties are the supervision of patients with AH, DM and other CNCDs and the identification of risk situations and referral to the responsible sectors, i.e. the health unit [47]

As part of their work routine, agents must make home visits at least once a month to each family living in their area. The number of visits per household varies depending on the health conditions of its inhabitants[47] .

During the visits, they must register and update the registration forms, under the supervision and monitoring of the nurse, assigned to the basic health unit of their reference, whose basic duties are to systematically coordinate, monitor, supervise and evaluate the work of the CHWs, the scheduling of home visits and the coordination and updating of the family registration forms[47] .

Replacing a CHA is only appropriate in situations where they no longer live in the area where they work, take on another activity that compromises the workload needed to carry out their activities, fail to fulfil their commitments and duties, generate conflict or rejection in their community and for private reasons, when the CHA themselves request their leave[47] .

As for the health team's professional staff, 19 (47.5%) reported alterations, with the doctor being mentioned by the majority (52.7%), followed by the nurse (21.0%).

Because it is a multifactorial disease, hypertension involves guidelines aimed at various objectives and will be effectively treated with the support of different health professionals. Multiple objectives require different approaches, and a multi-professional team provides this differentiated action, increasing the success of controlling hypertension and other cardiovascular risk factors[5] . What's more, hypertension poses the challenge of integrating different areas in order to advance knowledge and define the best clinical and therapeutic approach strategies for hypertensive individuals .[95]

It is of fundamental importance for multi-professional teams with different backgrounds to work on health education. Different perspectives on the same issue lead to better learning for the entire health team and, consequently, for patients, who are better orientated and have a greater chance of adhering to treatment and controlling their BP. The work of the multi-professional team can give patients and the community enough motivation to overcome the challenge of adopting attitudes that make antihypertensive actions effective and permanent[5] .

Of the total number of participants, 35 (87.5 per cent) reported not finding it difficult to monitor and treat their hypertension; the rest reported difficulties with the low-sodium diet, the doctor's presence in the health unit, scheduling medical appointments and obtaining orders and carrying out tests.

In the study carried out in São Paulo-SP, the main difficulty reported by the interviewees in the treatment of AH was the adoption of a low-sodium diet, followed by the difficulty of practising physical activity[98] .

In another study carried out in the municipality of Jequié-BA, which aimed to analyse adherence/abandonment to treatment in a group of hypertensive patients, the difficulties reported by the interviewees were the delay or lack of patient care (37.1%), the lack of medication (26.5%) and instructions on non-drug treatment (18.4%) and the inadequacy of the health professional-patient relationship (18%)[113] .

These difficulties are worrying because the obstacles that patients encounter in treating AH, such as changes in eating habits and regular physical activity, also apply to other associated diseases such as obesity, dyslipidaemia and diabetes[98] .

With regard to knowledge about hypertension and its implications, 17.5% of the participants mentioned some doubts about the disease. The origin of hypertension, its consequences and how physical activity should be practised were the doubts raised. However, although 82.5% of the participants reported having no doubts about hypertension, 45% reported having BP levels > 140/90 mmHg.

In a study carried out in the state of Paraíba[110] , 45.26 per cent of those interviewed said they had no doubts about the treatment of AH. Among those who reported having doubts, controlling the timing and dosage of medication, eating habits and whether or not physical activity was recommended were the most frequently mentioned.

The study carried out in São Paulo-SP[108] highlighted the association between knowledge of the disease and BP control. The satisfactory knowledge expressed by hypertensive patients was not related to BP control. This may indicate that the hypertensive patients in the study sample, despite expressing knowledge of important aspects of the disease and treatment, have not made sufficient changes to their lifestyle to achieve BP control.

We need to differentiate between knowledge and level of information. The literature shows that knowledge is more than knowing how to reproduce information, as it presupposes changes in attitudes, behaviour and lifestyle habits[72] . Knowledge alone does not guarantee changes in attitudes and behaviour; however, the right to information and mechanisms for this knowledge to be incorporated by any individual, regardless of their social situation, must be guaranteed .[114]

The hypertensive population must be aware of all the aspects inherent in the disease and its treatment. Clarification about the absence of specific symptoms, its chronicity, the types of treatments and the importance of long-term adherence to them, and the complications that can compromise vital organs when BP is not controlled, are essential aspects that hypertensive patients should be made aware of. Knowledge through educational processes is an unquestionable factor in properly following the treatment of hypertension and preventing its complications[89] .

Health education aims to make patients aware of the need to change their lifestyle, as well as understanding and knowing about the treatment and encouraging participatory behaviour[98] .

It is up to the multi-professional health team to search for up-to-date knowledge and innovative teaching strategies for the development of educational activities, and for users to commit to following the established therapy[72] . The health team's instructions to patients and their families should be clear, simple and properly recorded in the patient's medical records, avoiding disagreements between records and reports .[98]

For the educational process to be effective, it is necessary to know the individual's attitude towards the disease. It is also necessary for hypertensive patients to participate fully in their treatment, as most of the time they have the capacity to understand and collaborate, interacting with health professionals in the management of the health-disease process. The patient's customary health practices, values and perceptions in relation to the disease and treatment are different from those thought up by health professionals, since they are two different sociocultural, linguistic and psychological groups. It is therefore necessary to know and consider popular health practices in order to improve the effectiveness of care[115] .

When it came to evaluating the care and follow-up provided by health professionals at their unit, 6 (15.0%) interviewees reported that the service was excellent, 20 (50.0%) that it was good, 11 (27.5%) that it was regular and 3 (7.50%) that it was poor.

In the study carried out in the municipality of Jequié-BA, the evaluation of the work carried out by the health centre with hypertensive patients showed that 12.5% of the participants reported excellent, 31.0% good, 38.7% fair and 17.8% poor[113] .

Social control, as a legally established principle of the SUS, implies the possibility for users to intervene in health services, both in proposing policies and actions and in finalising their implementation. In this sense, its strengthening within the SUS and the encouragement of community participation, particularly in primary health care, presuppose the conception of the user as co-responsible for the management of the health system and with the competence to evaluate it, as well as to intervene and modify it[116].

The user thus stands out as the main qualifier of the health system by expressing their preferences, expectations, satisfaction or dissatisfaction with the methods, circumstances and results of care[117]. It is also considered that the quality of care is determined by the result, translated into the achievement of health and user satisfaction[116].

The user's role as a protagonist in the health system has a direct impact on improving the relationship between them and the service. It is essential to know how they evaluate the service, their opinion of the care provided and their level of satisfaction, in order to rethink professional practices or intervene in the way services are organised, with a view to improving them[116, 118].

The opinion of the user allows health actions to be adjusted and directed and expresses an indicator of the quality of the services provided. A positive evaluation of a service that doesn't fully meet the recommended health care standards may represent a passive and uncritical stance on the part of the user, possibly associated with low socioeconomic status, lack of knowledge of their rights, demonstrating the need for integration and participation in continuing education actions that make them more critical and reflective about the service they receive[101].

When asked for their opinion and suggestions about the health service where they were registered and monitored, the interviewees complained about the high turnover and lack of doctors in the health units, the difficulty in following up treatment and monitoring appointments and tests, and suggested hiring more doctors. They also mentioned the need for more frequent presence of CHWs at home.

The validity of prescriptions for longer and the prior scheduling of medical appointments were other suggestions mentioned, as they believed this would establish a greater commitment to attending appointments. Some hypertensive patients mentioned their share of responsibility for failures in their treatment, such as lack of attendance at appointments and meetings or failure to follow treatment. They also expressed the need for better care from the health team as a whole and more humanised care, where users could be heard in their doubts.

Access and reception are essential elements of care for achieving greater effectiveness in the individual's state of health and resolving problems related to basic health services. Access to health is linked to living conditions, nutrition, housing, purchasing power and education, encompassing accessibility to services, the difficulties faced in obtaining care, the treatment received by the user, the prioritisation of risk situations, urgencies and emergencies, the responses obtained to individual and collective demands and the possibility of scheduling appointments in advance. Welcoming consists of humanising the relationship between health service workers and users. It is understood as the attitude of the worker to put themselves in the user's shoes to feel what their needs are and, as far as possible, meet them or direct them to the place in the system that is capable of responding to those demands[118] .

CHAPTER 6

CONCLUSIONS

In view of the proposed objectives and the desire to learn a little about the reality of hypertensive patients in the municipality of the study in relation to some aspects related to human biology, the environment, lifestyle and the organisation of health services, the study obtained the following results:

6.1   Identification data

Of the 40 hypertensive patients who met the inclusion criteria, 57.5% were female, 55.5% were aged between 51 and 60, 65.0% were married and the average number of children was 2.4 ($\pm$1.3).

6.2   Human biology data

The average number of years since medical diagnosis of hypertension was 7.4 ($\pm$ 7) years, and 95.0% had been taking antihypertensive medication for an average of 4.4 ($\pm$ 4.3) years. Drug treatment was reported by 95.0% of the participants, 57.5% of whom used a combination of two, three or four drugs.

Adherence to this treatment as instructed by the doctor was reported by 85.0% of the participants and 55.0% reported BP levels < 140/90 mmHg

Among the main risk factors for the development and worsening of hypertension, the most cited were cardiovascular family history (85.0%), overweight/obesity (52.5%) and a sedentary lifestyle (42.5%). Complications resulting from AH were reported by 25.0%, with tachycardia and AMI standing out.

6.3   Environmental data

A family income of two to three minimum wages was reported by 50.0 per cent of the interviewees and the average number of people who depended on this income was 3.4 ($\pm$ 1.9).

The highest level of education was found in the same proportion (45.0%) of individuals with complete and incomplete first and second degrees, respectively. The majority of participants (57.5%) were active at work.

6.4   Lifestyle data

Given the importance of certain factors in BP control, the habit of eating a low-sodium diet was mentioned by 82.5% of the participants, who reported restricting sodium. None of the participants were able to say how many grams of sodium they consumed a day. Of those who were on a low-sodium diet, 56.3% reported that it was not the PACS doctor who had given them advice.

Of the participants, 60.0 per cent reported not using alcohol and 10.3 per cent reported using cigarettes for an average of 36.6 years, but were unwilling to mention the number of cigarettes per day.

The practice of physical activity was confirmed by 57.5% of the sample, with walking being the most cited exercise, 45.0% reported that they measured their BP at the pharmacy and 30.0% at the health unit.

Of those interviewed, 62.5 per cent reported changes in their habits and lifestyle to control BP, with salt and alcohol reduction being the most frequently cited.

6.5 Data on the organisation of health services

Of the population interviewed, 77.5 per cent confirmed that they only used public health services to treat their hypertension and that 85.0 per cent of the cases were diagnosed at a public health institution.

The majority (92.5%) said that they were followed up by the PACS doctor to treat their hypertension, and of the 34 who answered about the frequency of these consultations, 50.0% reported twice a year.

The initial drug treatment after the diagnosis of hypertension was reported by 67.5% of hypertensive patients and the acquisition of a prescription for antihypertensive drugs was informed by the majority, who sought it at the health unit; 20.5% mentioned that the CHA took the prescription to their home and 97.5% reported acquiring antihypertensive drugs at the Municipal Pharmacy.

Even though only one health centre provided continuing education activities for registered and monitored hypertensive patients, 56.3% reported not taking part due to lack of time and incompatible work schedules. The frequency of visits by CHWs to the homes of those interviewed varied from once a month (46.2%) to at least once every six months, and 75.0% reported that there was no replacement for the health worker when they were on holiday or on medical leave.

Of the total number of participants, 82.5% reported having sufficient knowledge about SAH and 50.0% reported that the care and follow-up provided by the health professionals at their health centre was good.

When asked about the quality of care and follow-up provided by the health professionals at their unit, many interviewees complained about the turnover and lack of doctors, and suggested hiring more professionals; they also called for an improvement in the care provided by the health team as a whole.

CHAPTER 7

FINAL CONSIDERATIONS

This study was an attempt to build up an overview of hypertension in the PACS of a municipality, in search of answers that could help improve care for hypertensive patients, from a health promotion perspective. The results presented made it possible to create a scenario of the reality studied and raised some reflections, even given the limited sample size used.

Analysing the data obtained from the consolidated SIAB[62, 119] , the prevalence of SAH in the municipality's PACS in 2011 was approximately 11.0%. In the municipality as a whole it was 13.0% and in 2012 it fell to around 7.0%. These results may indicate underestimated rates, which are not in line with the reality of this chronic disease and the prevalence figures currently found in Brazil.

The outdated and inconsistent number of hypertensive patients from the PACS found in the SIAB in 2011, as well as the figure obtained by active search, added to the decreasing prevalence of the disease in the municipality from 2011 to 2012, reinforce that the losses in the municipality's information system database generate the need to redo the old records. The lack of infrastructure in health units, such as more modern computers and software to prevent data loss, could be one reason for the situation found in the system's records, even though a probable lack of use of the information system has been proven.

In practice, this reality of feeding the database into the municipality's system is not in line with what the Ministry of Health has proposed for the programme, in terms of producing reports and helping teams, basic health units and municipal managers to monitor their work and evaluate the quality of the service. This information system should be seen as a tool for evaluating and planning the activities carried out and not just as a way of filling in information for the pure and simple purpose of receiving federal incentives.

PACS is a health programme that incorporates the SUS principle of universality. However, the data from the study showed that the fact that hypertensive patients are included in the programme may guarantee access to healthcare, but it does not ensure continuity of treatment and follow-up, due to the turnover and lack of healthcare professionals, especially doctors. Knowledge about the disease and its inherent care can also be jeopardised by the lack of periodic educational activities in the units, which could give voice to the expectations of hypertensive patients to seek solutions to their doubts, mistakes, slips, fears and complaints.

The lack of answers to some of the questions on the data collection form, especially those relating to lifestyle data and the organisation of health services, may initially demonstrate the fragility of the hypertensive individual/health system relationship. This may reflect a lack of involvement between the parties that could increase mutual trust, since the health service would provide guidance, monitoring and treatment of the disease and the hypertensive individual would demonstrate, through attitudes and results, their involvement with the treatment and monitoring of the disease. A second justification could have been the length of the interview form which, in an attempt to cover as many aspects of hypertension as possible, became long and tiring for the interviewees. And finally, the lack of responses related to lifestyle data, when hypertensive individuals were asked about their routine, health care and lifestyle habits, could reveal the hypertensive patients' share of responsibility and commitment to their health.

Although this research cannot make immediate contributions to changes in the health service, it has highlighted some weaknesses that could guide decision-making with a view to improving care for those involved. It is believed that its results could provide support for defining the needs and priorities of the municipality's PACS and, in general, the actions to be developed. Among these are prior scheduling of appointments, humanisation of care, the possibility of greater access and adherence to treatment for hypertensive patients, the creation and development of educational actions in health promotion, prevention of complications and treatment of hypertension, monitoring the participation of hypertensive patients in educational activities, medical or nursing appointments, as a way of monitoring their participation in the unit's activities, monitoring the progress of the disease, increasing the number of annual medical consultations, guaranteeing the acquisition of medication prescriptions after reassessment of the hypertensive patient's condition and access to the health service by including hypertensive patients who are not included in the municipality's information system records, in order to improve the conditions for their treatment and follow-up.

Although all these actions can promote the empowerment of hypertensive individuals registered and monitored by the PACS, above all valuing their effective participation in controlling the disease and changing their lifestyle habits, the question remains: would the results of the study have been different if the target had been hypertensive individuals registered with the municipality's PSF?

REFERENCES

1.	Lalonde M. A new perspective on the health of Canadians: a working document: Health and Welfare Canada. Ottawa. 1974.
2.	Brandão AA, Magalhães M, Ávila A, Tavares A, Machado C, Campana E, et al. VI Brazilian Guidelines on Hypertension. Arq Bras Hipertens. 2010;95(11-17).
3.	Brazil MdS. Surveillance, control and prevention of chronic non-communicable diseases: NCDs in the context of the Brazilian Unified Health System Ministry of Health. Ministry of Health - Brasília : Pan American Health Organisation. 2005( ):80.
4.	Paiva Dd, Bersusa AAS, Escuder MML. Evaluation of care for patients with diabetes and/or hypertension by the Family Health Programme in the Municipality of Francisco Morato, São Paulo, Brazil. Cad Saúde Pública. 2006;22(2):377-85.
5.	Cardiology SBd. V Brazilian guidelines for arterial hypertension. Hipertensão. 2006;9(4).
6.	Malta DC, Castro AMd, Gosch CS, Cruz DKA, Bressan A, Nogueira JD, et al. The National Health Promotion Policy and the physical activity agenda in the context of the SUS. Epidemiologia e Serviços de Saúde. 2009;18(1):79-86.
7.	Boing AC, Boing AF. Systemic arterial hypertension: what the Brazilian health registration and information systems tell us. Rev Bras Hipertens. 2007;14(2):84-8.
8.	Franco R. Revista Hipertensão - Abstracts Brazilian Society of Hypertension. 2012;Vol 1 Supplement.
9.	Cesarino CB, Cipullo JP, Martin JFV, Ciorlia LA, Godoy MRPd, Cordeiro JA, et al. Prevalence and sociodemographic factors in hypertensive patients in São José do Rio Preto-SP. Arq Bras Cardiol. 2008;91(1):31-5.

10.	Miranzi SdSC, Ferreira FS, Iwamoto HH, Pereira GdA, Miranzi MAS. Quality of life of individuals with diabetes mellitus and hypertension monitored by a family health team. Texto e Contexto Enfermagem. 2008;17(4):672.
11.	WHO. The world health report 2002. Reducing risks, promoting healthy life. Available at: http://wwwwhoint/whr/2002/en/whr02_enpdf Accessed on: 29/03/2013. 2002;Geneva.
12.	Costa H, Solla J, Almeida M, Curitiba D. Inquérito domiciliar sobre comportamento de risco e morbidade referida de doenças e agravos não transmissíveis. Rio de Janeiro: National Cancer Institute. 2004.
13.	Passos VMdA, Assis TD, Barreto SM. Hypertension in Brazil: prevalence estimates from population-based studies. Epidemiologia e Serviços de Saúde. 2006;15(1):35-45.
14.	VIGITEL B. Surveillance of risk and protective factors for chronic diseases by telephone survey. Secretaria de Vigilância em Saúde Departamento de Análise de Situação de Saúde Estatística e Informação em Saúde Ministério da Saúde. 2012;1ª ed; Serie G; Brasília - DF.
15.	PAD. Bulletin of the PAD-MG Household Sample Survey: Healthy living habits. João Pinheiro Foundation, Statistics and Information Centre. 2012;Year 1; n. 4; Belo Horizonte p. 1 - 80.
16.	Castro RAAd, Moncau JEC, Marcopito LF. Prevalence of systemic arterial hypertension in the city of Formiga, MG. Arq Bras Cardiol. 2007;88(3):334-9.
17.	Barreto SM, Passos VMA, Firmo JOA, Guerra HL, Vidigal PG, Lima-Costa MFF. Hypertension and clustering of cardiovascular risk factors in a community in Southeast Brazil: the Bambuí Health and Ageing Study. Arq Bras Cardiol. 2001;77(6):576-81.
18.	Lessa Í, Magalhães L, Araújo MJ, Almeida Filho Nd, Aquino E, Oliveira MM. Hypertension in the adult population of Salvador (BA)-Brazil. Arq Bras Cardiol. 2006;87(6):747-56.
19.	Goldman L, Ausiello D. Cecil Medicina - Tratado de Medicina Interna Ed Elsevier Ltda. 2010;23a ed(Rio de Janeiro):3720.
20.	Irwin S, JS T. Cardiopulmonary Physiotherapy. Ed Manole. 2003;3rd ed (São Paulo).
21.	Powers S, E H. Physiology of Exercise. Ed Manole. 2009;6th ed. (São Paulo).
22.	Figuiredo D, Azevedo A, Pereira M, de Barros H. Deknition of Hypertension: The Impact of Number of Visits for Blood Pressure Measurement [61]. Rev Port Cardiol. 2009;28(7-8):775-83.
23.	Chobanian AV, Bakris GL, Black HR, Cushman WC, Green LA, Izzo JL, et al. Seventh report of the joint national committee on prevention, detection, evaluation, and treatment of high blood pressure. Hypertension. 2003;42(6):1206-52.
24.	Fauci AS, Longo DL, Kasper DL, Hauser SL, Jameson JL, Loscalzo J. Harrison's Internal Medicine. 18ª ed Rio de Janeiro: Artmed Editora. 2012.
25.	Gerais M. Adult health care: Hypertension and Diabetes. State Department of Health SAS/MG Belo Horizonte
Available	at	http://www.saude.mg.gov.br/publicacoes/linha-guia/linhas-guia/LinhaGuiaHiperdia.pd Accessed on 22/06/2012. 2007.
26.	Carvalho MVd, Jardim PCB, Sousa ALL. The influence of hypertension on quality of life. Arq Bras Cardiol. 2013;100(2):164-74.
27.	Kohlmann JOea. III Brazilian Consensus on Arterial Hypertension. Arq Bras Endocrinol Metab [online] Accessed: 02/03/2013. 1999;43(4):257-86.
28.	Brazil MdS. Cadernos de Atenção Básica 7 - Hipertensão Arterial Sistêmica - HAS and Diabetes Mellitus - DM: Protocolo. Brasília. 2001;96p.
29.	Malachias MVB, Souza WKSBd, Lotemberg AMP, Guimarães AC, Negrão CE, Forjaz CLdM, et al. Non-drug treatment and multiprofessional approach. Brazilian Journal of Nephrology. 2010;32:22-8.
30.	Appel LJ, Brands MW, Daniels SR, Karanja N, Elmer PJ, Sacks FM. Dietary approaches to prevent and treat hypertension a scientific statement from the American Heart Association. Hypertension. 2006;47(2):296-308.
31.	Rosemberg J, Rosemberg AMA, Moraes MA. Nicotine: universal drug. Available at: http://wwwincagovbr/tabagismo/publicacoes/nicotinapdf Accessed on: 02/04/2013. 2005:240.
32.	Santos ZMdSA, Lima HdP, Oliveira FBd, Vieira JS, Frota NM, Nascimento JCd. Adherence of hypertensive users to drug therapy. Revista da Rede de Enfermagem do Nordeste-Rev Rene. 2013;14(1).
33.	Brasil MdS. Evaluation of the Plan to Reorganise Care for Hypertension and Diabetes Mellitus in

Brazil. Ministry of Health Pan American Health Organization Series C Projects, Programmes and Reports. 2004;Brasília - DF.

34.   Leavell H, Clark E. Preventive medicine Ed McGraw-Hill. 1976;Rio de Janeiro.

35.   Becker D. In the bosom of the family: breastfeeding and health promotion in the Family Health Programme. Rio de Janeiro. 2001.

36.   Czeresnia D, Freitas CMd. Promoção da saúde: conceitos, reflexões, tendências; Health promotion: concepts, reflections, tendencies. 2003;Rio de Janeiro:174.

37.   Heidmann I, Almeida MCP, Boehs AE, Wosny AdM, Monticelli M. Health promotion: historical trajectory of its conceptions. Texto Contexto Enferm. 2006;15(2):352-8.

38.   Castro A, Serrano M. SUS: ressignificando a promoção da saúde: Ed. Hucitec; 2006.

39.   Ferreira M, Castiel L, Cardoso MdA, editors. Health Promotion: between conservatism and change
.   Brazilian Congress of   Sports   Sciences;
2007:   Available at   :
http://www.cbce.org.br/cd/resumos/023.pdf Accessed on: 21/06/2012.

40.   Brazil MdSSdPdSPPdS.   The   health   promotion
charters.   Available at   :
http://dtr2001saudegovbr/editora/produtos/livros/pdf/02_1221_Mpdf   Accessed   on: 17/18/2011.
2002;Brasília(Série B. Textos Básicos em Saúde):56.

41.   Buss PM, Carvalho AId. Development of health promotion in Brazil in the last twenty years (1988-2008). Ciência & Saúde Coletiva. 2009;14(6):2305-16.

42.   Raddatz A, Scholze AdS, Júnior C, Silveira P. Discourse analysis of the National Health Promotion Policy Revista Brasileira em Promoção da Saúde. 2012;24(3):191-8.

43.   Buss PM. Health promotion and quality of life. Ciênc saúde coletiva. 2000;5(1):163-77.

44.   Carvalho Ad. Principles and practice of health promotion in Brazil. Cad Saúde Pública, Rio de Janeiro. 2008;24(1):4-5.

45.   Escorel S, Giovanella L, Mendonça MHM, Senna MdCM. The Family Health Programme and the construction of a new model for primary care in Brazil. Rev Panam Salud Pública. 2007,21(2):164-76.

46.   Brazil C. Constitution of the Federative Republic of Brazil: Constitutional text promulgated on 5 October 1988, as amended by Constitutional Amendments Nos. 1/92 to 52/2006 and by Constitutional Amendments for Revision Nos. 1 to 6/94 2006. Senado Federal, Subsecretaria de Edições Técnicas. 1998;Brasília.

47.   Brazil   MdSSE.   Community   Health   Agents   Programme   (PACS).   Available   at: http://bvsmssaudegovbr/bvs/publicacoes/pacs01pdf Accessed on: 03/09/2011. 2001;Brasília:40.

48.   Viana AL, Dal Poz MR. Health system reform in Brazil and the Family Health Programme. Physis. 1998;8(2):11-48.

49.   Dal Poz MR. The community health worker: some reflections. Interface-Comunic, Saúde, Educ. 2002;6(10):75-94.

50.   Pereira H, Limongi JE. Community health workers: duties and challenges. Hygeia. 2011;7(12).

51.   Institutional IT. Family Health Programme. Rev Saúde Pública. 2000;34(3):316-9.

52.   Brasil MdS. Municipal health management: basic texts. Ministry of Health Brasília; 2001.

53.   Toscano CM. National campaigns to detect chronic non-communicable diseases: diabetes and hypertension. Ciênc Saúde Coletiva. 2004;9(4):885-95.

54.   Institutional IT. Plan for the Reorganisation of Hypertension and Diabetes Mellitus Care. Rev Saúde Pública. 2001;35(6):585-8.

55   Brazil   MdSSdVeSSdAàS   National   Health   Promotion   Policy.   Available   at: http://portalsaudegovbr/portal/arquivos/pdf/pactovolume7pdf Accessed on: 01/10/2011. 2006;Brasília(Series B.Textos básicos):60.

56.   Gil A. How to prepare research projects. Publisher: Atlas. 1996,São Paulo.Ed. 3ª.

57.   IBGE.   Brazilian   Institute   of   Geography   and   Statistics   (IBGE)   Available   at: http://wwwibgegovbr/home/estatistica/populacao/estimativa2011/tab_Municipios_TCUpdf   Accessed   on: 09/01/2013. 2011.

58.   IBGE. Brazilian Institute of Geography and Statistics (IBGE). Available at:

http://wwwibgegovbr/cidadesat/xtras/perfilphp?codmun=314800 Accessed on: 09/02/2013. 2013.

59.   PatosdM. Patos de Minas City Hall. Available at : http://wwwpatosdeminasmggovbr/acidade/negociosphp Accessed on: 06/03/2011. 2011.

60.   CNES. National Register of Health Establishments - CNES Net - Secretariat of Health Care; Ministry of Health/ DATASUSDavailable at: http://cnesdatasusgovbr/Lista_Es_Municipioasp?VEstado=31&VCodMunicipio=314800&NomeEstado=MINAS%20GERAIS Accessed 03 April 2013. 2009.

61.   DATASUS. Health Information Booklet - General information. Available at: ftpdatasusgovbr Accessed on 13/07/2012. 2009.

62.   SMS. Consolidation of families registered in 2011 Secretariat of Health Care/ DAB - DATASUS Municipal Secretariat of Health Primary Care Information System (SIAB). 2012(version: 6.6):1-5.

63.   Statute. Statute of Children and Adolescents. Law No. 8069, of 13 July 1990 Subchefia para Assuntos Jurídicos/Casa Civil/Presidência da República. 1990(Available at : http://www.planalto.gov.br/ccivil_03/leis/l8069.htm Accessed 10/05/2013).

64.   Statute. Law No. 10.741, of 10 October 2003. Statute of the Elderly. Federal Senate. Available at: http://wwwplanaltogovbr/ccivil_03/leis/2003/l10741htm Accessed on: 28/03/2012. 2003;Brasília.

65.   Brazil MdS. SIAB: basic care information system manual. Secretaria de Assistência à Saúde, Coordenação de Saúde da Comunidade. Available at: http://18928128100/dab/docs/publicacoes/geral/manual_siab2000pdf Accessed on 29/09/2012. 1998;Brasília:98.

66.   Faria CCdC, Morraye MdA, Santos BMdO. Diabetics from a health promotion perspective. Rev Bras em Promoção da Saúde. 2013;26(1):26-35.

67.   Baldan S. The leprosy patient: an approach from the perspective of health promotion. [Dissertation] Unifran. 2010.

68.   Sampaio F, Melo R, Rolim I, Siqueira R, Ximenes L, Lopes M. Evaluation of health promotion behaviour in patients with diabetes mellitus. Acta Paul Enferm. 2008;21(1):84-8.

69.   Brazil MdSCNdS. Resolution 196, of 10 October 1996: guidelines and regulatory standards for research involving human beings. National Health Council, National Committee for Ethics in Research on Human Beings. Available at: http://conselhosaudegovbr/resolucoes/reso_96htm Accessed on: 08/0/2011. 1996;Brasília.

70.   Jardim PCBV, Gondim MdRP, Monego ET, Moreira HG, Vitorino PVdO, Souza WKSB, et al. Hypertension and some risk factors in a Brazilian capital. Arq Bras Cardiol. 2007;88(4):452-7.

71.   Magnabosco P. Health-related quality of life of individuals with hypertension who are members of a community group. Ribeirão Preto - SP: [Dissertation] Ribeirão Preto School of Nursing/ USP. ; 2007.

72.   Oliveira K. Knowledge and attitudes of users with type 2 diabetes mellitus and hypertension in a Basic Health Unit in Ribeirão Preto. Ribeirão Preto: University of São Paulo, Ribeirão Preto School of Nursing. 2009.

73.   Cotta RMM, Batista KCS, Reis RS, Souza GAd, Dias G, Castro FAFd, et al. Socio-sanitary profile and lifestyle of hypertensive and/or diabetic users of the Family Health Programme in the municipality of Teixeiras, MG. Ciênc Saúde Coletiva. 2009;14(4):1251-60.

74.   Tavares D. Health conditions of elderly diabetics. Ribeirão Preto Nursing School University of São Paulo. 2001;Ribeirão Preto - SP(Thesis: doctorate).

75.   Mion DJ, Pierin A, Bambirra A, Assunção J, Monteiro J. Hypertension in employees of a University General Hospital Rev Hosp Clin Fac Med Univ São Paulo. 2004;59(6):329-36.

76.   Baldissera VDA, Carvalho MDdB, Pelloso SM. Adherence to non-pharmacological treatment among hypertensive patients at a school health centre. Revista Gaúcha de Enfermagem. 2009;30(1):27.

77.   Veras R. Contemporary population ageing: demands, challenges and innovations. Rev Saúde Pública. 2009;43(3):548-54.

78.   Taveira LF, Pierin AMG. Can socioeconomic status influence the characteristics of a group of hypertensive patients? Revista Latino-Americana de Enfermagem. 2007;15(5).

79.   Lima SGd, Nascimento LSd, Santos Filho CNd, Albuquerque M, Victor EG. Systemic arterial

hypertension in the emergency department: the use of symptomatic drugs as an alternative treatment. Arq Bras Cardiol. 2005;85(2):115-23.

80.   Gus I, Harzheim E, Zaslavsky C, Medina C, Gus M. Prevalence, recognition and control of systemic arterial hypertension in the state of Rio Grande do Sul. Arq Bras Cardiol. 2004;83(5):424- 8.

81.   Mochel EG, de Andrade CF, de Almeida DS, Tobias AF, Cabral R, Cossetti RD. Evaluation of the treatment and control of systemic arterial hypertension in public health patients in São Luís (MA). Revista Baiana. 2007:90.

82.   Nobre F, Pierin AM, Mion Junior D. Adherence to treatment: the challenge of hypertension. Ed: Lemos Editorial. 2001;São Paulo - SP.

83.   WHO WHO. Innovative care for chronic conditions: structural components for action: world report. World Health Organisation Brasilia; 2003.

84.   Brazil MdS. Strategic action plan for tackling chronic non-communicable diseases (NCDs) in Brazil 2011-2022. Ministry of Health Secretariat of Health Surveillance Department of Health Situation Analysis; 2011.

85.   Monteiro FPM, Vitor AF, de Oliveira Lopes MV, de Araujo TL, Vasconcelos JDP, Morais HCC. Profile of therapeutic follow-up conditions in patients with arterial hypertension. Escola Anna Nery Revista de Enfermagem, Available at: http://wwwredalycorg/articulooa?id=127719099006 Accessed on 07/02/2013. 2011;15(2):251-60.

86.   Verri V, Cunha AB, Tessarolo LE, Carneiro RC, Romeo LJM. Reduction of Myocardial Ischaemia after Treatment with Simvastatin in Patients with Chronic Coronary Artery Disease [73]. Portuguese journal of cardiology. 2004;23(9):1089-105.

87.   Oliveira CJd, Moreira TMM. Characterisation of the non-pharmacological treatment of elderly people with hypertension. Revista da Rede de Enfermagem do Nordeste-Rev Rene. 2012;11(1).

88.   Fuchs FD, Moreira LB, Moraes RS, Bredemeier M, Cardozo SC. Prevalence of systemic arterial hypertension and associated factors in the urban region of Porto Alegre: a population-based study. Arq Bras Cardiol. 1995;63(6):473-9.

89.   Pierin A, Mion J, Fukushima J, Pinto AR, M. K. The profile of a group of hypertensive people according to knowledge and severity of the disease. Rev Esc Enf USP. 2001:35(1):11-8.

90.   Piati J, Felicetti CR, Lopes AC. Nutritional profile of hypertensive patients followed up by Hiperdia in a Basic Health Unit in a city in Paraná. Rev Bras Hipertens. 2009;16(2):123-9.

91.   Romero AD, Silva MJd, Silva ARVd, Freitas RWJFd, Damasceno MMC. Characteristics of an elderly hypertensive population cared for in a family health unit. Revista da Rede de Enfermagem do Nordeste-Rev Rene. 2012;11(2).

92.   Brazil MdSSdPdS. Plano de reorganização da atenção à hipertensão arterial e ao diabetes mellitus: manual of hypertension and diabetes mellitus: Brazil. Ministry of Health; 2002.

93.   SBD SBdD. Treatment and monitoring of diabetes mellitus: Guidelines of the Brazilian Diabetes Society Ed: Diagraphic. 2007;Rio de Janeiro - RJ.

94.   Piccini RX, Victora CG. Systemic arterial hypertension in an urban area in southern Brazil: prevalence and risk factors. Rev Saúde Pública. 1994;28(4):261-7.

95.   Pereira APR, Barreto MIC, Oliveira S. O perfil dos usuários hipertensos cadastrados e acompanhados por uma Unidade de Saúde da Família de um município do interior do leste mineiro [monografia]. Caratinga University Centre. 2008;Caratinga - MG.

96.   Brasil tA, A.C. Controle da hipertensão arterial: uma proposta de integração ensino-serviço: Ministério da Saúde; 1993.

97.   Martins IS, Marucci MdFN, Velásquez-Meléndez G, Coelho LT, Cervato AM. Atherosclerotic cardiovascular diseases, dyslipidemias, hypertension, obesity and diabetes mellitus in a population from a metropolitan area in the Southeast Region of Brazil. III-Hypertension. Rev Saúde Pública. 1997;31(5):466-71.

98.   Figueiredo NN, Asakura L. Adherence to antihypertensive treatment: difficulties reported by hypertensive individuals. Acta Paulista de Enfermagem. 2010;23(6):782-7.

99.   Contiero AP, Pozati MPS, Challouts RI, Carreira L, Marcon SS. Elderly with arterial hypertension: difficulties in monitoring in the Family Health Strategy. Revista Gaúcha de Enfermagem. 2009;30(1):62.

100.   MacGregor GA, He FJ. How far should salt intake be reduced? Hypertension 2003;42(6):1093-9.

101.	Guandalini V. Estratégia saúde da família: avaliação dos cuidados em saúde e nutrição aos adultos diabéticos e hipertensos, Matão/SP. Available at: http://www2fcfarunespbr/Home/Pos-graduacao/AlimentoseNutricao/valdete-regina-guandalini---dopdfTese Accessed on: 16/ 10/2013. 2013.

102.	WHO. International guide for monitoring alcohol consumption and related harm. World Health Organisation. 2000;Geneva:51-5.

103.	Jardim P, Monego E, Sousa A. The non-drug approach to patients with hypertension In: Pierin AMG Hipertensão arterial: uma proposta para o cuidado. Ed: Manole. 2004;Barueri.

104.	Fuchs FD, Moreira WD, Ribeiro JP. Antihypertensive efficacy of aerobic physical conditioning: a critical analysis of experimental findings. A critical analysis of experimental findings. Arq bras cardiol. 1993;61(3):187- 90.

105.	GravinaTaddei CF, Ramos LR, Moraes JCd, Wajngarten M, Libberman A, Santos SC, et al. Multicenter study of elderly patients in outpatient clinics of cardiology and geriatric Brazilian institutions. Arq Bras de Cardiol. 1997;69(5):327-33.

106.	Sousa L, Souza R, Scochi M. Hipertensão arterial e saúde da família: atenção aos portadores em município de pequeno porte na região sul do Brasil. Arq Bras Cardiol 2006;87(1).

107.	Brazil MdSSdAàSDdAB. Política Nacional de Atenção Básica - Série Pactos pela Saúde Ministério da Saúde. 2006;Brasília - DF (4):60.

108.	Strelec M, Pierin AM, Mion Jr D. The influence of knowledge about the disease and attitude towards taking medication on hypertension control. Arq Bras Cardiol. 2003;81(4):349- 54.

109.	Coelho EB, Moysés Neto M, Palhares R, Cardoso M, Geleilete TJM, Nobre F. Relationship between attendance at outpatient appointments and blood pressure control in hypertensive patients. Arq Bras Cardiol. 2005;85(3):157-61.

110.	Lucena M, Medeiros J, Dantas R. Knowledge of hypertension patients about their treatment. FIEP Bulletin On-line Special Edition Available at: http://wwwfiepbulletinnet Accessed: 01/10/2013. 2011;81(1).

111.	Lopes HF, Barreto-Filho JAS, Riccio GMG. Non-drug treatment of arterial hypertension. Rev Soc Cardiol Estado de São Paulo. 2003;13(1):148-55.

112.	Silva M, Santos M. Activity profile of community health agents linked to the Family Health Programme in the northern area of Juiz de Fora. Rev APS. 2005;8(2).

113.	Mascarenhas CHM, Oliveira MML, Souza MS. Adherence to treatment in the hypertensive group in the Joaquim Romão-Jequié/BA neighbourhood. Rev Saúde Com. 2006;2(1):30-8.

114.	Knuth A, Bielemann R, Silva G, Borges T, Del Duca GF, Kremer M, et al. Adults' knowledge about the role of physical activity in the prevention and treatment of diabetes and hypertension: a population-based study in Southern Brazil. Cad Saúde Pública. 2009;25(3):513-20.

115.	Péres DS, Magna JM, Viana LA. People with hypertension: attitudes, beliefs, perceptions, thoughts and practices. Rev Saúde Pública. 2003;37(5):635-42.

116.	Jorge MSB, Guimarãesb JMX, Vieirac LB, de Paivad FDS, Rocha D, Pintof SAGA. Quality assessment of the Family Health Programme in Ceará: user satisfaction. Revista Baiana. 2007:258.

117.	PAHO/WHO. Renewing Primary Health Care in the Americas: Position Paper of the Pan American Health Organisation/World Health Organisation (PAHO/WHO). 2007;Washington, D.C: PAHO,.

118.	Ramos DD, da Silva Lima MAD. Health care access and receptivity to users in a unit in Porto Alegre, Rio Grande do Sul, Brazil. Cad saúde pública. 2003;19(1):27-34.

119.	SMS. Consolidation of registered families for 2012. Secretaria de Assistência a Saúde/ DAB - DATASUS Secretaria Municipal de Saúde Sistema de Informação de Atenção Básica (SIAB). 2013(version: 6.6.1).

Model Sheet A
(Front)

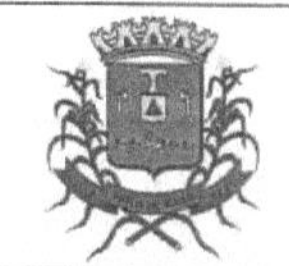

PREFEITURA DE PATOS DE MINAS	UF
SECRETARIA MUNICIPAL DE SAÚDE	

FICHA A

SISTEMA DE INFORMAÇÃO DA ATENÇÃO BÁSICA
SAÚDE DA FAMÍLIA

ENDEREÇO: ___ Nº ___ BAIRRO ___ CEP ___ — ___

MUNICÍPIO ___ SEGMENTO ___ ÁREA ___ MICRO-ÁREA ___ FAMÍLIA ___ DATA ___

1 - Cadastro da família

Nº	PESSOAS COM IDADE DE 15 ANOS E MAIS NOME	PARENTESCO	DATA DE NASCIMENTO	IDADE	SEXO	ALFABETIZADO? QUE NÍVEL	OCUPAÇÃO	DOENÇA OU COND. REFERIDA
			___/___/___					
			___/___/___					
			___/___/___					
			___/___/___					
			___/___/___					
			___/___/___					
			___/___/___					
			___/___/___					
			___/___/___					
			___/___/___					
			___/___/___					

Nº	PESSOAS COM IDADE DE 15 ANOS E MAIS NOME	PARENTESCO	DATA DE NASCIMENTO	IDADE	SEXO	ALFABETIZADO? QUE NÍVEL	OCUPAÇÃO	DOENÇA OU COND. REFERIDA
			___/___/___					
			___/___/___					
			___/___/___					
			___/___/___					
			___/___/___					
			___/___/___					
			___/___/___					
			___/___/___					
			___/___/___					
			___/___/___					

SIGLAS PARA INDICAÇÃO DAS DOENÇAS E/OU CONDIÇÕES REFERIDAS			
ALC - Alcoolismo	DRC - Usuário de drogas		
BRQ - Bronquite	EPI - Epilepsia		
CHA - Chagas	GES - Gestação		
DEF - Deficiência física	HAN - Hanseníase		
DME - Distúrbio mental	OB - Obesidade		
DES - Desnutrição	DRC - Tuberculose		

2 - Situação de moradia e saneamento

2.1 Tipo de domicílio

☐ Tijolo/Alvenaria

☐ Adobe

☐ Taipa revestida

☐ Taipa não revestida

☐ Madeira

☐ Material aproveitado

☐ Outros

2.2 N° de cômodos

2.3 Trab. Água domicílio

☐ Filtração

☐ Fervura

☐ Cloração

☐ Sem tratamento

2.4 Abast. de água

☐ Rede pública

☐ Poço ou nascente

☐ Outros

2.5 Energia elétrica

☐ Sim ☐ Não

2.6 Esgoto sanitário

☐ Rede pública

☐ Fossa

☐ Céu aberto

2.7 Destino do lixo

☐ Coletado

☐ Queimado/enterrado

☐ Céu aberto

3 - Outras informações

Alguém da família possui Plano de Saúde

☐ SIM

☐ NÃO

N° de pessoas cobertas

Nome do Plano

Em caso de doença procura

☐ Hospital ☐ Farmácia

☐ Unidade de saúde

☐ Benzedeira ☐ Outros: _____

Participa de grupos comunitários

☐ Cooperativa ☐ Não

☐ Grupo religioso

☐ Associações

☐ Outros: _____

Meios de transportes

☐ Ônibus ☐ Carroça

☐ Caminhão

☐ Carro

☐ Outros: _____

Meios de comunicação que mais utiliza

☐ Rádio ☐ Televisão ☐ Outros: _____

Observações

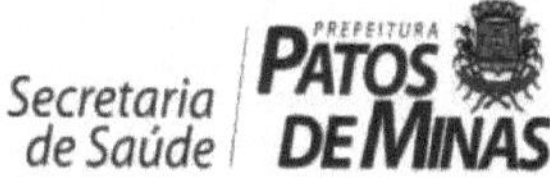

DECLARAÇÃO

Declaro ter lido e concordar com o parecer ético emitido pelo Comitê de Ética em Pesquisa da Universidade de Franca, conhecer e cumprir as Resoluções Éticas Brasileiras, em especial a Resolução CNS 196/96. A Prefeitura Municipal de Patos de Minas está ciente de suas co-responsabilidades como instituição colaboradora do presente projeto de pesquisa, e de seu compromisso no resguardo da segurança e bem-estar dos sujeitos de pesquisa nela recrutados, dispondo de infra-estrutura necessária para a garantia de tal segurança e bem-estar.

Patos de Minas, 21 de dezembro de 2011.

____
Janaina Maria Silva Araújo Souza
Secretária de Saúde do Município de Patos de Minas

Statement of final approval from CEPE

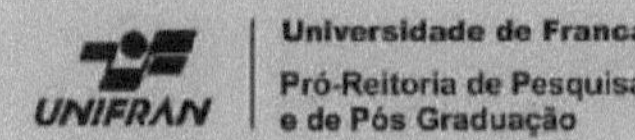 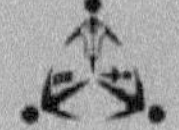 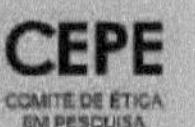

PROTOCOLO DE ENTREGA (relatório final)

Declaro que recebi de **Nair Caetano Domingos** o relatório final do projeto de pesquisa nº **0087.0.393.393-11**, do qual é a pesquisadora responsável, na data de 25/11/2013.

Por ser verdade firmo o presente,

Daniela Tasso Teixeira

Secretária do CEPE/UNIFRAN

Av. Dr. Armando Salles Oliveira, 201 – CEP 14404-600 – Franca – SP - Brasil – Fone: (16) 3711 - 8904 – Fax (16) 3711 - 8829 – E-mail: cepe@unifran.br

APPENDIX A

INFORMED CONSENT FORM
(National Health Council, Resolution 196/96)

Name of participant: ____

Identity document: _________________________________ Date of birth ___ /___ / ______________

CPF no:____

Address: ____ Nº _________ Apt: __________

Neighbourhood: _______ postcode: _____________ CITY:_______________________________

Telephone(s): ____

I, the above-qualified person, AGREE to participate in the research "THE PATIENT OF SYSTEMIC ARTERIAL HYPERTENSION FROM A HEALTH PROMOTION PERSPECTIVE", coordinated by the researcher in charge ProE. DE. Branca Maria de Oliveira Santos and conducted by Nair Caetano Domingos, a student/researcher on the "Master's in Health Promotion" course at the University of Franca. They explained to me that this research is justified by the risks that hypertension entails, as well as its evolution. It will be important to know the conditions of my living environment, my habits and lifestyle and the health care I receive in order to guide my choices, which will determine the level of health and quality of life I will have in the future. The results could provide elements for developing individual and collective actions within the health system to improve health and the services provided.

When I was invited to take part, it was explained to me that the objectives of the research are:

1. to characterise the living and health conditions of individuals with systemic arterial hypertension, registered with the Community Health Agents Programme (PACS) - in the health units of the Sebastião Amorim I, Guanabara, Jardim Paraíso and Ipanema neighbourhoods, in order to assess and learn about the clinical conditions, risk factors, problems and difficulties faced in treating and monitoring the disease;

2. the data collection procedure consists of an interview form that will be applied by the researcher, in a single moment, during a previously scheduled home visit, at a time when I am available. The interview will consist of questions about my identification data, clinical data, human biology data (about my illness), the environment in which I live, my lifestyle and the organisation of the health services where I receive care. That this interview will not cause any harm to my health; that I will be guaranteed clarification of my doubts as many times as I deem necessary, before and during the course of the research and that my participation is voluntary, and that I have the right to refuse to take part for any reason or to withdraw at any time from the study, without any prejudice or penalty, even if the research does not offer me any kind of risk or harm;

3. I am aware that the expected benefits of taking part in this study are: contributing to scientific research; effectively taking part in a study that could enlighten me about my living conditions and health and, in general, those of the hypertensive patients registered with the PACS in my neighbourhood; understanding my pathology, how and where I need to improve in order to reduce the potential risks it could bring me; knowing what other diseases could arise if I don't really take care of my habits, lifestyle and living conditions and health, as well as contributing to always improving the health care provided to me in our unit;

4. explained to me that the researcher will guarantee absolute confidentiality with regard to my identity, that I will be guaranteed anonymity and that my name and information will not be revealed under any circumstances. The results of the study may be presented and publicised at events and in scientific journals, without, however, divulging my name, under their responsibility and the penalties laid down in Brazilian law;

5. I know that my participation is free of charge and does not imply any kind of remuneration, aid or subsidy. I also know that I have no obligation to pay for my free participation;

6. i am aware that i may withdraw from participation at any time, without this implying liability or cancellation of the services offered by this institution;

65

7. I will have the right to contact the researcher and the Research Ethics Committee of the University of Franca at any time to clarify any doubts that may arise during the research, and I therefore have the right to information;

8. Finally, I will receive a copy of this document with the names and contact telephone numbers of the researcher and the Research Ethics Committee of the University of Franca.

I declare that I FREELY agree to participate in this research, as I have been fully informed by the researcher and understand the objectives, risks and benefits of my participation in this study.

Signature of participant (Research Subject)

Patos de Minas, ________ of ________________________________2012.

Name of Researcher Responsible: Nair Caetano Domingos
Tel: (34) 8849 - 0252 / (34) 9117 - 8311
E-mail: naircae2@yahoo.com.br
University of Franca Research Ethics Committee: (16) 3711-8904.
E-mail: cepe@unifran.br. Address: Av. Dr. Armando Salles Oliveira, 201 CEP: 14404-600, Pq. Universitário, Franca, São Paulo.

RESEARCHER'S DECLARATION

I DECLARE, for research purposes, that I have drawn up this Free and Informed Consent Form (FICF), complying with all the requirements contained in Chapter IV of Resolution 196/96 and that I have obtained, in an appropriate and voluntary manner, the free and informed consent of the above-qualified research subject to carry out this research.

Patos de Minas, ______of _____________________________ 2012.

Signature of the researcher responsible (name in full)

APPENDIX B

INTERVIEW FORM

1) Identification Data:
Health unit (PACS): ____
Date:___/___/ _____
1.1) Name (initials) ____
1.2) Sex: M ( ) F ( ) Date of birth: ______________/_____/____
1.3) Age: ___________
1.4) Marital status No. of children
1.5) Address____

1.6)   Contact telephone numbers ____

2)   Human Biology Data:

2.1)   Colour: ( )White ( )Black ( )Yellow ( )Brown ( )Mulatto

2.2)   How long has it been since you were diagnosed with hypertension? _______________________
How high is your blood pressure normally? (last measurement) _______________________________

2.3)   ( ) Yes ( ) No For how long? ____
Which one(s)?____
<u>Other associated medicines: </u>____

2.4)   When you feel well or when your blood pressure is close to normal, do you stop taking your blood pressure medication? Yes ( ) No ( )
If not, why?____
How many days can you go without the medication? _______________________

2.5)   Risk factors for developing SAH:
( )DM ( ) DMID ( ) DMNID
( ) smoking ( ) sedentary lifestyle
( ) overweight/obese ( ) dyslipidaemia
( ) Family history. - Which one(s)?

HAS	DM	Angina	IAM	STROKE	Renal Insuff. Renal	Sudden Death
( ) Yes	( ) Yes	( ) Yes	( ) Yes	( ) Yes	( ) Yes	( ) Yes
( )No	( )No	( )No	( )No	( ) No	( )No	( )No
( ) I don't know	( ) I don't know	( ) I don't know	( ) I don't know	( ) I don't know	( ) I don't know	( ) I don't know

( )Father	( )Father	( )Father	( )Father	( )Father	( )Father	( )Father
( )Mum	( )Mum	( )Mum	( )Mum	( )Mum	( )Mum	( )Mum
( ) Sister	( ) Sister	( ) Sister	( ) Sister	( ) Sister	( ) Sister	( ) Sister
( ) Other	( ) Other	( ) Other	( ) Other	( ) Other	( ) Other	( ) Other

2.6)   Complications arising from SAH:
( )AMI ( )Stroke ( ) Kidney disease ( ) Depression ( ) Tachycardia ( )Angina
( )other ____

3)   Environmental data

3.1)   Level of education:
(   ) illiterate   (   ) 2nd degree complete
(   ) 1st degree incomplete   (   ) higher education   incomplete
(   ) Completed first degree   () Completed   higher education
(   ) Incomplete secondary education   (   ) Vocational training

3.2)   Family income (in minimum wages = R$ 632.00)
( ) up to 1   ( ) 2 to 3( )   3 to 6( )   6 to 10(   ) over 10
- How many people depend on this income? _____________________________________

3.3)   Current work situation: ( ) active ( ) retired ( ) unemployed ( ) on leave
( ) Household ( ) Other ____

3.4)   If working: Place of work____

Working _________________ hours per week. Time in the job? _________________________________

3.5)   If retired or on leave, for how long? ____

4)   Lifestyle data

4.1)   Do you eat a low-sodium diet?
( )Yes ( )No.
If not, why?____

If yes: was she advised by the PACS doctor?
( )Yes ( )No.
If not: who guided you?
( )health agent and/or PACS nurse ( )nutritionist ( )family member
( )acquaintances ( )books/magazines ( )radio/TV programmes ( )internet
How many grams of sodium do you eat a day? ____

4.2)   Consumption of alcoholic beverages: Yes ( ) No ( )
If yes. _________________________________ TypeFrequency ____________________
Quantity: ( )g of alcohol/day ____

4.3)   Smoking: Yes ( ) No ( )
If yes: Type: ____
Frequency: ____________ Time: ______________ Quantity: ____________________________

4.4)   Physical exercise: Yes ( ) No ( )
If yes: Type____
Frequency: ________________ Duration: ___________ How long ago? ____________________
If not, why? ____

4.5)   Have you changed your habits and lifestyle to control your blood pressure?
( )Yes ( )No.
If yes. What?____
4.6)   Where do you "measure" your blood pressure?
( )PACS ( )pharmacy ( )at home ( )neighbour ( ) I don't monitor my blood pressure
( ) Other ____

4.7)   How often do you "measure" your blood pressure?
( )daily ( )weekly ( )   monthly ( )annually
( )every six months   ( ) 3x/week   ( )almost never

5)   Data related to the Organisation of Health Services:

5.1)   Do you have private health insurance? ( ) Yes ( ) No

5.2)   In which health centre was you diagnosed with hypertension? ____________________________

5.3)   Are you followed up by the doctor at the health unit (PACS) to treat the disease?
( )Yes ( )No.
If yes. How often: ____
If no. The doctor who accompanies you is ( )insured, ( )private or ( ) I don't follow up.

5.4)   When you received a medical diagnosis of hypertension, what action did you take?
( ) drug treatment was started immediately
( )was orientated and encouraged to adopt changes in their habits and lifestyle before "going on" the

medication.
( ) Both.

5.5)   How do you get your antihypertensive prescription?
( ) I'm going to the petrol station to pick her up.
( )A family member goes to the petrol station to pick them up.
( )The health worker takes the prescription to your home.

5.6)   Who supplies your antihypertensive medication?
( )Municipal Pharmacy ( )Family ( ) You ( )Other_______________________________

5.7)   In 2011, were there any meetings, lectures or discussion groups on SAH at the health centre where you
receive care, to clarify your doubts and advise you on healthy lifestyle habits?
( )Yes ( )No.
If yes. How often? ____
Did you attend these educational activities? ( )Yes ( )No.
If no. Reason:____

If yes. Importance____

Who does the guidance?____

5.8)   How often does the health worker visit you at home?
( )one visit/month ( )one visit every 1 month and ^ ( )one visit every 2 months
( ) one visit every 3 months
( )Other ____

5.9)   If your health worker doesn't turn up due to holidays or a doctor's certificate, does someone replace
them?
( )Yes ( )No

5.10)   In 2011, were you accompanied by the same PACS team (doctor/nurse/agents)? ( )Yes ( )No.
If not. What changes have taken place in this period?___________________________________

5.11)   Do you face any difficulties in monitoring and treating the disease?
( ) yes ( ) no. If yes, which ones?____

5.12)   Do you have any questions about the disease? Yes ( ) No ( )
If yes, which one(s)____

5.13)   How do you rate the care and follow-up provided by the health professionals - doctors, nurses and
community health workers at your health unit (PACS)?
( )great ( )good ( )fair ( )bad
Justify your answer:____

5.14)Do you feel limited because you have hypertension? ( )Yes ( )No.
If yes. Reason ____

5.15)
a)   What is your opinion of the health service where you are registered and monitored?

b)   What would you like to see changed in the care provided by this service?

Space reserved for comments by interviewee: ____

Date: ______//_____

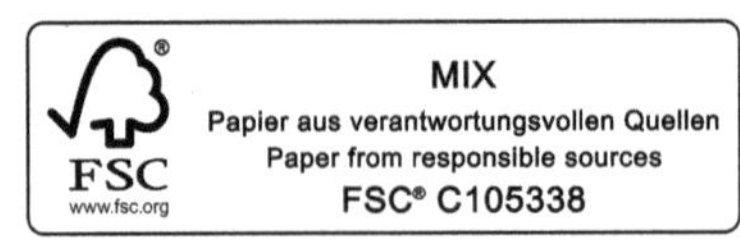

Printed by Books on Demand GmbH, Norderstedt / Germany